TAKING CHARGE

of High Blood
Pressure

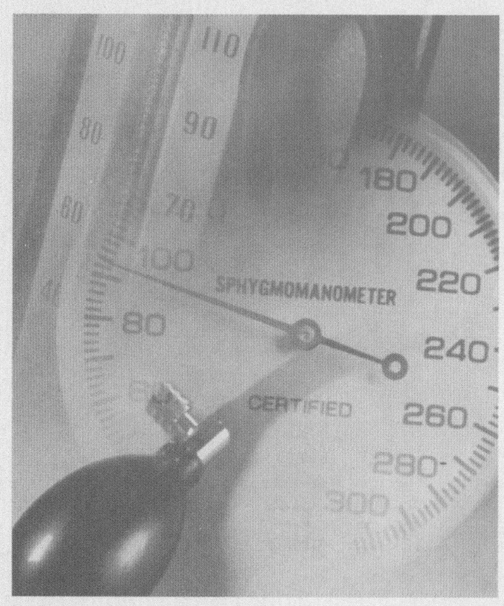
SPHYGMOMANOMETER
CERTIFIED

TAKING CHARGE

of High Blood Pressure

SUSAN PERRY

The Reader's Digest Association, Inc.
Pleasantville, New York/Montreal

Contents

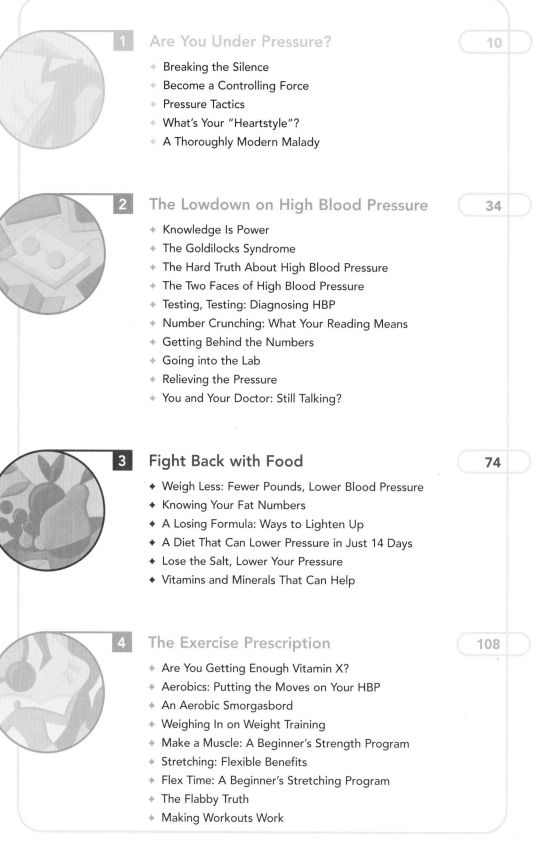

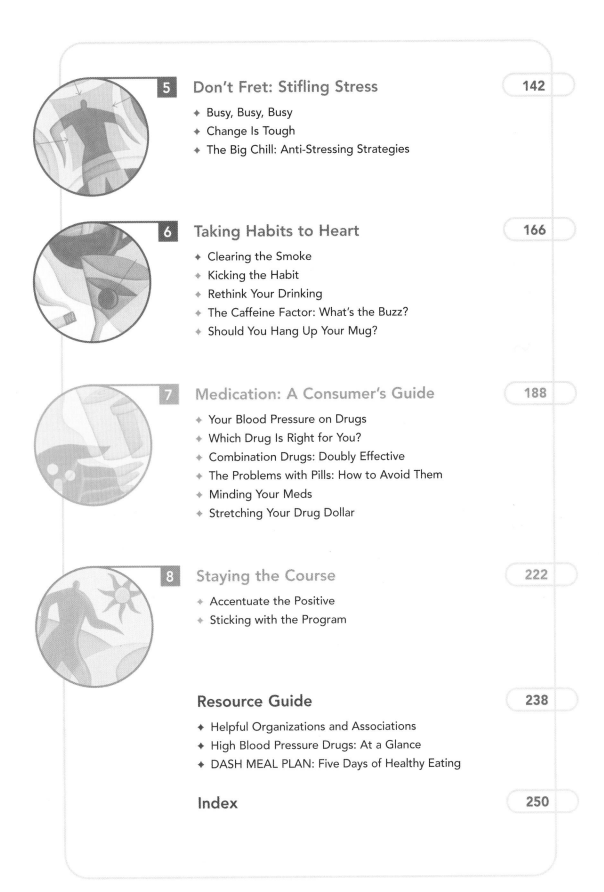

READER'S DIGEST PROJECT STAFF

Senior Editor
Wayne Kalyn

Production Technology Manager
Douglas A. Croll

Editorial Manager
Christine R. Guido

CONTRIBUTORS

Writer
Susan Perry

Design
Spinning Egg Design Group

Senior Designer
Martha Grossman

Illustrators
Tracy Walker (editorial)
Articulate Graphics (medical)

Indexer
Robert Elwood

MEDICAL CONSULTANT

William P. Castelli, MD,
Director of the Framingham
Cardiovascular Institute,
Framingham, Massachusetts

READER'S DIGEST HEALTH PUBLISHING

Editorial Director
Chris Cavanaugh

Art Director
Joan Mazzeo

Marketing Director
James H. Malloy

Vice President/General Manager
Shirrel Rhoades

READER'S DIGEST ASSOCIATION, INC.

Editor-in-Chief
Eric W. Schrier

President, North American Books and Home Entertainment
Thomas D. Gardner

Library of Congress Cataloging in Publication Data

Perry, Susan. 1950-
Taking charge of high blood pressure: start today strategies for combatting the silent killer / Susan Perry.

p. cm.
ISBN 0-7621-0351-5 (hardcover)
ISBN 0-7621-0393-0 (softcover)
1. Hypertension—Popular works.
I. Title
RC685.H8 P368 2001
616.1'32—dc21   2001031821

Address any comments about Taking Charge of High Blood Pressure to:
Reader's Digest
Editorial Director, Health
Reader's Digest Road
Pleasantville, NY 10570

To order additional copies of Taking Charge of High Blood Pressure, call
1-800-846-2100

Visit our website at:
www.rd.com

Printed in the United States of America
1 3 5 7 9 10 8 6 4 2

NOTE TO READERS

The information in this book should not be substituted for, or used to alter, medical therapy without your doctor's advice. For a specific health problem, consult your physician for guidance.

US 4049H/IC

About This Book

High blood pressure gets no respect, as Rodney Dangerfield often laments about his own sorry persona. Some 50 million people in the United States suffer from it, but only one-third take action to get it down to levels where it won't compromise their health or shorten their life. The condition does both with alarming regularity.

People with high blood pressure aren't solely to blame for their inaction. Survey results suggest that patients aren't aware of the implications of hypertension—a fancy word for high blood pressure—options for treatment, or how the disease is managed. In other words, the patient-doctor dynamic these days is so hurried and rushed that physicians don't have the time to provide a meaningful explanation of most chronic diseases during office visits. And as doctors know, an uninformed patient is an undertreated patient.

Taking Charge of High Blood Pressure will make sure that this won't happen to you. The book has an optimistic message—almost everyone can lower their blood pressure levels—and a practical game plan that enables you to do just that. The book essentially fills the knowledge gap and empowers you to lower your blood pressure numbers quickly and effectively.

You will learn everything you need to know about risk factors, how to make sure you are getting accurate BP readings and the correct diagnosis, thorough information about the latest treatments, and easy-to-follow strategies for working with your doctor.

This exceedingly helpful book takes a multiple-choice approach to treatment. In many cases, a one-two punch of diet and exercise can often deflate high blood pressure numbers. In others, treatment will require adding stress reduction to the mix as well as abandoning habits that you might not know are elevating your pressure: smoking for one, and excessive alcohol consumption for another. If all this "lifestyle medicine" doesn't do the trick, then medication most certainly will.

But more than anything, *Taking Charge of High Blood Pressure* urges and motivates you to take action—today, now. Every new day is another opportunity to take a stand against a deadly condition you can control and overcome.

Foreword

By the time people reach their 50s in the United States, half of them will have high blood pressure. The condition is a leading risk factor for strokes, heart attacks, kidney failure, and other vascular problems. At its heart, blood pressure is a numbers game. I

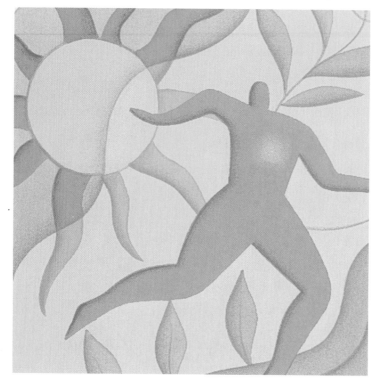

can't say it enough: Know your BP numbers. If they are too high or borderline high, do everything in your power to lower them. If they are optimal or normal, do everything you can to keep them that way.

But how did the medical community come to understand what the blood pressure numbers mean—which numbers mean trouble, which are ideal? It is a gift from the people of Framingham, Massachusetts, and the Framingham Heart Study. For over 50 years the good people of Framingham allowed researchers to put them under a microscope. Since 1948, physicians have been measuring Framingham residents' blood pressure numbers and other important statistics and examining them to find out who went on to have a heart attack, stroke, or other diseases.

The medical community learned volumes. For example, once your systolic pressure (the upper number) reaches 120 and your diastolic pressure (the lower number) hits 80, you start to pay a price for too high a blood pressure. And what happens if a person lowers his or her blood pressure? More than 40 trials have shown that the person dramatically reduces his or her risk for heart attack and stroke. In fact, we have a workable solution to prevent most of the vascular disease in the world. Are we taking advantage of it? Sadly, no.

Taking Charge of High Blood Pressure can help you right now. It will get you up to speed on the importance of your blood pressure numbers and help you assess what you can do to lower them. Hypertension is silent in most people until the day they have a stroke or heart attack. Those people waited too long to do something about their blood pressure. This book serves as your wake-up call.

"When it comes to blood pressure, people have to become the keeper of their own numbers."

If you know you have elevated blood pressure *Taking Charge of High Blood Pressure* can help to change your life for the better. Early on, you will learn about how many people develop high blood pressure. In America it has a lot to do with sloth and gluttony. You will also learn how diet—more vegetables and fruit, and less sodium—can change that. Exercise is another great help in lowering blood pressure numbers. Controlling stress as well as other lifestyle approaches are also critical to lowering your pressure.

People have to take a more active part in controlling their health. And when it comes to blood pressure, people have to become the keeper of their own numbers. You must learn what your blood pressure numbers are and how to maintain them in the ideal or optimal range, not just the average range. Understand that this book is not a substitute for your doctor, but it will help you understand what your doctor will do when you are diagnosed with high blood pressure and what you can do on your own to make it all work.

The number one cause of death in the U.S.—heart disease—could almost disappear if we really lowered our risk factor numbers for it, such as cholesterol and high blood pressure. You need to seize this opportunity to fashion a better lifestyle for yourself and for your loved ones. Start today. —William Castelli, MD

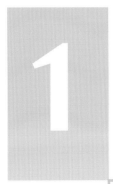

Are You Under Pressure?

If you were recently diagnosed with high

blood pressure, or if you have known about

the condition for a while but have been stead-

fastly ignoring it or only half-heartedly taking

steps to control it, consider this your wake-up

call. You can—and should—control your blood

pressure, and live a healthier and longer life.

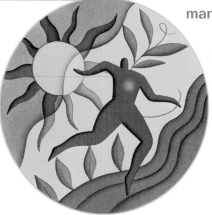

KEY CONCEPT High blood pressure is highly controllable—by you, in many cases. Although the condition is deadly if ignored, it is probably the easiest of all chronic diseases to manage.

Breaking the Silence

The first thing you should know about having high blood pressure—or hypertension, as it's known in medical-speak—is that you're not alone.

According to the World Health Organization, some 500 million to 1 billion people suffer from the condition around the world. Within the United States, as many as 50 million people can claim the condition as their own.

To put a face on that latter statistic, that means one out of four co-workers standing around the office coffee pot have high blood pressure, or, closer to home, one out of four people sitting around the Thanksgiving dinner table. (For people over 50, the number escalates to one in two.) Now for another statistic that might elevate the blood pressure numbers even of a yogi: One-third or more of the people with the condition don't know they have it.

No pain, no problem? Don't be quick to point an accusing finger at these in-the-dark hypertensives. Unlike arthritis or a bum back, high blood pressure rarely announces itself or shows any symptoms. You can have it for years and feel perfectly okay—until, that is, you suffer one of its very serious consequences, such as a stroke or heart attack. Doctors aren't being melodramatic when they call high blood pressure a "silent killer."

Which leads us to the second thing you should know about high blood pressure: If you've been diagnosed with it, you can consider yourself, in a way, very, very fortunate. At least you know you need to take steps to get your blood pressure down to normal levels. For you, staying healthy is a very real option.

> **Pressure Point:** High blood pressure isn't really a disease because it usually has no symptoms and therefore doesn't make you feel sick. But it is a risk factor —and a big one—for stroke, heart disease, aneurysms, as well as vision and kidney problems.

For those of you who *don't know* if your blood pressure is too high for your own good, it's time to "break the silence" and get your BP checked. Do it as soon as possible. Don't just assume everything is okay because you feel fine. Remember: Not knowing your blood pressure numbers can be dangerous—even fatal—to your health.

Become a Controlling Force

High blood pressure is a lifelong condition. Which means it can't be cured—not by a doctor, not by you. But don't worry: The good news is that the condition lends itself to self-treatment.

In fact, compared with all other chronic diseases, high blood pressure is probably the easiest to control. And control is as good as a cure because it reduces all of the health risks associated with the condition.

Many years ago, doctors often advised newly diagnosed hypertensives to quit their day job and to go into social hibernation—avoiding any activities that might be the slightest bit stressful. Today, fortunately, that advice is considered outmoded. No longer do you have to take a diagnosis of high blood pressure lying down! You can have the condition and continue to lead a full, active—and long—life.

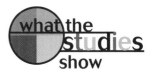
what the studies show

► *The National Institutes of Health confirms that untreated hypertension leads to widespread disability and premature death. It is estimated, for example, that a 35-year-old healthy white American male with normal blood pressure can expect to live to 75 years. However, with high blood pressure, his life expectancy is only 55 years.*

Go on the offensive. The key to living well with elevated blood pressure is getting it under control. By treating the condition aggressively—and that is the operative word—you can dramatically reduce its damaging effects. In fact, studies have shown that lowering blood pressure to normal levels can add at least one to five years to your life and perhaps many more.

Treatment is essential, however. You can't simply ignore your high blood pressure and hope it will go away. The strategy is straightforward: Seek the care of a medical professional who will work with you—not lecture you—on developing a take-charge treatment plan. Then comes the truly hard part: Following through with that plan. In almost every case, your success rests squarely on your own shoulders. After all you will be the one quarterbacking your plan day by day.

Do You Run a Risk?

Knowing the risk factors of high blood pressure is the first step in transforming you from a disinterested bystander into an active participant in your own health. Read the questions below and check off any that apply to you.

- Do you have family members (parents, brothers, sisters, grandparents) with high blood pressure?

- Are you overweight?

- Are you African American?

- Are you a man over the age of 35?

- Are you a woman past menopause?

- Do you smoke cigarettes or use smokeless tobacco?

- Do you regularly drink more than two alcoholic beverages per day?

- Are you sedentary?

- Do you take oral contraceptives?

If you answered "yes" to any of these questions, then you may be at risk for high blood pressure.

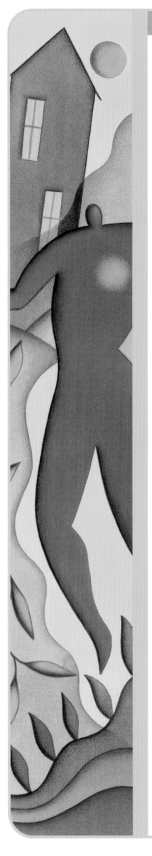

REAL-LIFE MEDICINE

Living Well with High Blood Pressure

Mark Tomlinson was stunned to learn his blood pressure was high—150/110 mm Hg—during his annual checkup. He was a fit 51, a relief-sculpture artist in River Falls, Wisconsin. His doctor said lifestyle changes might be enough to drive down the numbers; if not, medication would. Tomlinson asked about the medication's potential side effects and learned that sexual dysfunction was possible.

"That was a price I didn't want to pay," says Tomlinson. He had experienced erectile dysfunction (ED) during his first marriage; it was something he didn't want to go through again. He told his doctor that medication wasn't an option. What specifically were the lifestyle changes that needed to be made? His physician had two words for him: diet and exercise. Tomlinson agreed that he would make them. "I was willing to do whatever it took to turn this around."

True to his word, Tomlinson started drinking more water and reducing his salt, caffeine, alco-hol, and fatty food intake. He did tai chi, played tennis, and walked 1.6 miles in 21 minutes every morning. He meditated at sunrise, concentrating on breathing techniques that could slow his mind and pulse rate from 60 beats per minute to 45. Meditation, he says, also rolled over into prayer, which helped reduce stress that related to the time-pressured, business side of being an artist.

Tomlinson's efforts have paid off in the three years since the diagnosis. He does not use medication and his blood pressure is usually around 130/80. High blood pressure is in his family, so Tomlinson has no illusions that his hypertension is history. "I need to be diligent in my lifestyle choices, not push, push, push myself so." In practical terms, that means not letting his job cause too much stress in his life—fretting over meeting deadlines and such, and worrying that the work will continue to come his way.

"In the long run, I believe my high blood pressure episode will add years to my life and more satisfaction to my middle years."

> **"I was willing to do whatever it took to turn this around."**

High Blood Pressure: Kids' Stuff, Too

Doctors used to think that high blood pressure in children was almost always caused by other diseases, usually heart or kidney disease. But now they know this isn't so. Studies have shown that otherwise healthy children—including toddlers—can develop high blood pressure.

In fact, experts estimate that about 2 percent of children under the age of 18 in the United States have high blood pressure. African American children seem to be especially at risk. And the numbers are growing—mainly, say the experts, because kids are getting fatter. Today, about 11 percent of kids age 6 to 17 in the U.S. are overweight—a prime risk factor for HBP—more than double what the percentage was during the 1960s and 1970s.

Act now. Make sure your child's blood pressure is checked annually. Should your child be diagnosed with high blood pressure, his or her doctor will probably recommend a change in diet, more exercise, and perhaps some medication. Kids are given the same medication to control high blood pressure as adults, only in smaller doses.

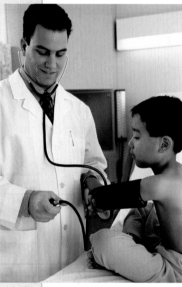

>**Pressure Point:** Researchers believe that we could reduce the number of cases of hypertension by 20 to 50 percent if people with borderline blood pressure readings would do what they need to do now to lower it.

Remember: Thousands of people with high blood pressure have lowered their BP to safe levels and others have helped prevent the condition in the first place. All it takes is learning how and then turning that knowledge into action. In the end, an uninformed patient is an undertreated patient, more likely to develop a stroke or other cardiovascular problem.

Pressure Tactics

Taking charge of your high blood pressure will require you to reevaluate many of your daily habits and then make changes. Take heart, though: Even a small drop in BP will lower your risk for major problems.

There's no getting around it: You'll need to commit yourself to a healthy lifestyle, and you must make that commitment day in and day out for the rest of your life. If you stop treatment because you "feel fine," you risk having your blood pressure shoot back up to harmful levels.

Change is good. Experts recommend that people with high blood pressure introduce 10 "action steps" into their daily routine. Most of these recommendations—such as not smoking, getting your weight down, and exercising more—are no-brainers. You've undoubtedly heard these suggestions before. One or two of them, such as eating more potassium-rich foods—and getting enough of the minerals calcium and magnesium—may be more surprising to you. In addition, studies have shown that a diet high in fruits and vegetables, whole grains, and low-fat or no-fat dairy foods can make a dramatic difference in lowering BP and keeping it low.

In fact, many people have lowered their blood pressure so significantly through lifestyle changes alone that they never need to take high blood pressure medication.

But whether you've known for years that you should be taking these steps to get healthier, or whether you're just now learning about them, don't delay taking action any longer. Your health depends on it. And chances are you won't need years of treatment to begin seeing the benefits, because even the smallest drop in blood pressure can greatly improve your chances of avoiding serious problems.

Drop your pressure, lift your spirits. Now, before you start groaning about the seemingly impossible task of embracing a new slate of healthful habits (and shedding unhealthful ones in the process), consider this: Evidence from the 1997 Hypertension Optimal Treatment (HOT) trial, one of the largest high blood pressure studies ever conducted, revealed that aggressively taking steps to lower blood pressure is more likely

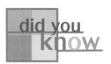

did you know

▶ *If not treated and controlled, high blood pressure can cause:*

➤ *Stroke*

➤ *Heart attack*

➤ *Kidney problems*

➤ *Eye problems*

➤ *Death*

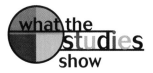

what the studies show

▶ *Research in the journal* Hypertension *revealed that there is actually a "salt gene." The study showed that people with one of the three forms of the so-called salt gene (angiotensinogen) were most likely to develop high blood pressure. Fortunately, this same group responded best to a reduced-sodium diet.*

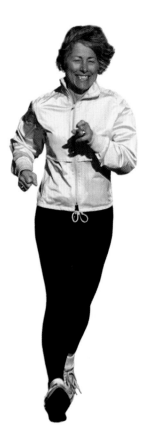

to lift your mood than to deflate it. In the study, people who successfully took charge of their high blood pressure scored better in virtually all aspects of psychological well-being than those whose blood pressure remained high. In other words, small victories in lowering your pressure a little gives you the confidence that you can lower it even more.

Here, then, are snapshots of the 10 steps that will help lower your pressure. You'll find detailed information about each of them in later chapters.

Know your numbers

Only by monitoring your blood pressure will you know whether you're maintaining it at a healthy level. So you'll need to play medical accountant and track your BP by checking it regularly and writing down the results. Did you know, for instance, that blood pressure is constantly changing: Simply getting up from a chair spikes it upward; sleep, as you would guess, drops it. In Chapter 2, you'll learn what you should do to make sure you get accurate blood pressure readings and what the numbers mean.

Pare the pounds

People who are overweight are two to six times more likely to develop high blood pressure than people who aren't over-weight. If you are lugging around more pounds than you should (more than half of the people in the United States are), you'll need to shed some of them. Then, once you arrive at a healthier weight, you'll need to develop a strategy to keep them off. *Taking Charge of High Blood Pressure* has you covered. In Chapter 3 you'll learn the latest techniques from experts to help you part with pounds—for good.

Move it, lose it

The studies are clear: People who are physically active are 20 to 50 percent less likely to have high blood pressure than those who are inactive. So if you're a long-standing couch potato, you'll need to pry yourself from your cushioned perch and shake it up. Don't know how to get started? Chapter 4 is a great place to start.

4 A DASH of nutrition

Thanks to the landmark 1997 study called DASH—Dietary Approaches to Stop Hypertension—we now know that you can eat your way to lower blood pressure. In a nutshell, the DASH diet is high in fruits, vegetables, and low-fat dairy foods and low in fat and saturated fat— not exactly a reflection of the typical American diet. Chances are, you'll need to make some adjustments to your eating habits. For help in revamping your cooking style and food choices, turn to Chapter 3, and for five days' worth of tasty meals, turn to the *Resource Guide* at the back of the book.

5 Shake off the salt

Past studies have shown that some people with high blood pressure—many experts believe it's less than half of those with the condition—are "salt-sensitive," or likely to see their blood pressure fall if they restrict how much salt they eat. New research has revealed, however, that everyone—even people without high blood pressure—could experience a healthy reduction in blood pressure by cutting back on salt. Chapter 3 will show you how, and reveal surprising sources of sodium-rich foods and tasty salt-free solutions.

6 Pack in the potassium

People who eat a lot of foods rich in the mineral potassium tend to have lower blood pressure. Potassium helps accomplish that by creating a healthy balance of sodium in your cells. In fact, potassium is the third most abundant mineral in the body. If your present diet isn't potassium-rich—full of legumes (beans, peas, and lentils), vegetables, and fruit—you'll need to find ways of making it so. Again, Chapter 3 will provide a laundry list of potassium-rich sources and practical information about how to enhance your diet with this miracle mineral, as well as with calcium and magnesium.

Small Changes, Big Impact

If your lifestyle changes only lower your blood pressure a small amount, you will be immensely better off. Here's what making a few basic changes could do for you and the American public in terms of reducing systolic blood pressure (the first number in a blood pressure reading):

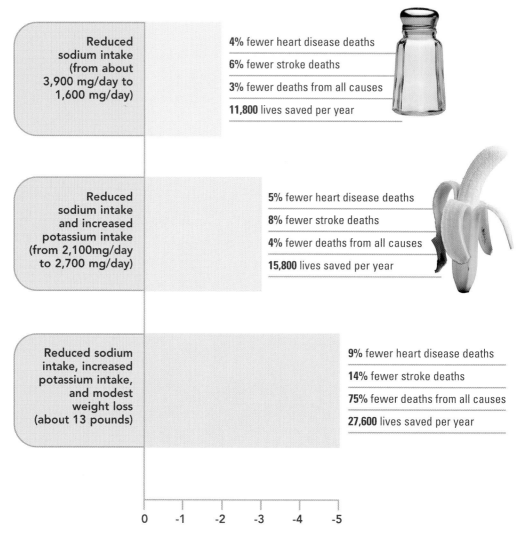

Reduced sodium intake (from about 3,900 mg/day to 1,600 mg/day)
- **4%** fewer heart disease deaths
- **6%** fewer stroke deaths
- **3%** fewer deaths from all causes
- **11,800** lives saved per year

Reduced sodium intake and increased potassium intake (from 2,100mg/day to 2,700 mg/day)
- **5%** fewer heart disease deaths
- **8%** fewer stroke deaths
- **4%** fewer deaths from all causes
- **15,800** lives saved per year

Reduced sodium intake, increased potassium intake, and modest weight loss (about 13 pounds)
- **9%** fewer heart disease deaths
- **14%** fewer stroke deaths
- **75%** fewer deaths from all causes
- **27,600** lives saved per year

0   -1   -2   -3   -4   -5

Reductions in Systolic Blood Pressure (mm Hg)

SOURCE: *Hypertension*, November 1989

7 Stress less

Got stress? Who doesn't. A stressful event or an emotional encounter can shoot your blood pressure sky high. Experts are less certain, however, about whether ongoing stress from the travails and annoyances of modern life—crowded cities, congested highways, long work hours, money worries, and road, phone, and other "rages"—raises blood pressure over the long term. But, until the final verdict is in, you'd be wise to take steps to reduce the stress in your life or, at the very least, to find better ways of coping with life's sometimes relentless demands. Chapter 5 will give you several de-stressing approaches for calming mind and body.

> **Pressure Point:** Being anxious or depressed doubles your risk of having high blood pressure. Scientists aren't sure why. It may be because mood has a physiological effect on blood vessels. Or it may be because anxiety and depression often lead to behaviors, such as overeating, smoking, and alcohol abuse, that can send blood pressure soaring.

8 Butts out

Add elevated blood pressure to the long list of smoking's nasty negatives. So if you smoke, you'll need to quit. Yes, yes, quitting is hard, but the health benefits are huge. Chapter 6 will tell you about all of them. If you're a nonsmoker, don't even think about starting.

You'll also need to stay away from other people's smoke, which can raise your blood pressure and harm your health in other ways. Did you know that living or working with a smoker can actually be deadlier than smoking itself? Secondhand smoke isn't filtered, and, as a result, contains much higher concentrations of tar,

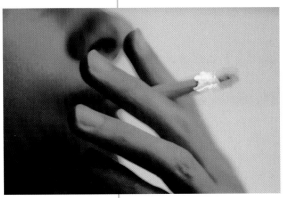

nicotine, and more than 4,000 other compounds. For the latest info on successful stop-smoking strategies—for yourself or someone you care about—see Chapter 6.

9 Go easy on alcohol

Drinking alcohol elevates blood pressure, particularly in people who are overweight or older. But here comes the paradox: Some studies have also shown that people who drink alcohol moderately (one or two drinks per day) tend to have lower blood pressure and less heart disease than abstainers.

If you already drink alcohol, you'll need to limit your consumption (if you haven't already) to no more than two drinks daily. But if you don't drink, there's no need to start now. You can take many other, more healthful actions (action steps one through eight for starters) to lower your blood pressure and protect your heart. Chapter 6 will help you rethink your drinking.

> **Pressure Point:** High blood pressure is the culprit behind 7 percent of all premature deaths worldwide. That percentage will grow as more societies give up their walking shoes for automobiles and their low-salt, low-fat native cuisine for salty, high-fat fare.

10 Say yes to drugs

People with moderately high blood pressure can often control the condition by adopting—and sticking with (the hard part)— lifestyle changes alone. But for more severe cases of high blood pressure or for those stubborn cases that don't respond to healthier habits, drug treatment is usually necessary. If you fall into one of these categories, you'll need to take medications as prescribed by your doctor. (For an at-a-glance list of all high blood pressure drugs, please turn to the *Resource Guide* at the back of the book.)

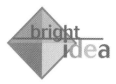

bright idea

▶ *Take advantage of every free blood pressure screening you come across—at the mall, at your local pharmacy, at your workplace, or wherever else one might be offered. (Just make sure the screening is done by a nurse or a qualified practitioner.) Write down your blood pressure numbers as well as the date and time that each reading was taken. A multitude of readings will give you a better idea of whether your blood pressure is too high than an annual one-time reading in a doctor's office.*

The problem is, which one will work for you? There are nine classes of high blood pressure medication—and each comes in different brand names and subtypes and in a variety of doses. Confused yet? To help you through this medicinal morass, see Chapter 7.

More Carrots to Lower BP

Okay. Just in case warding off a heart attack, stroke, blindness, or kidney failure isn't a compelling enough reason for you to give up your daily buttered muffin fix or to actually walk rather than drive those few blocks to your local library or grocery store, then check out the following laundry list of other health benefits you can enjoy by adopting many of the action steps:

> You'll have more endurance and energy because your heart won't have to work as hard.

> You'll experience less stress, tension, and anxiety.

> Your mood will improve.

> You'll sleep better.

> Your body will be stronger and more flexible, which means you'll find it easier to move about and do your daily tasks.

> Your mind will stay sharper.

> You'll greatly lower your risk of getting a host of other chronic conditions, including diabetes, certain types of cancer, and osteoporosis.

Now for the Things You Can't Control (Or Can You?)

Age

Question: The older you get, the greater your risk for developing high blood pressure, right? Answer: Only if you live in an industrialized country. People who live in areas of Africa and other parts of the world where physical labor and eating low-salt,

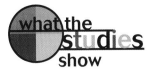

what the studies show

● *High blood pressure may be a risk factor for neovascular (wet) age-related macular degeneration (ARMD), the leading cause of irreversible blindness in the United States. Those with wet ARMD were four times more likely to have elevated diastolic (the second number in a blood pressure reading) than those with dry ARMD.*

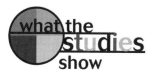

what the studies show

▶ *High blood levels of insulin, often caused by obesity (especially significant accumulation of fat in the abdomen), can indirectly elevate blood pressure levels. Insulin heightens the activity of the sympathetic nervous system and also causes sodium retention by the kidneys, both of which raise blood pressure. If you suffer from insulin resistance syndrome, also called Syndrome X, talk to your doctor about the consequences on your blood pressure.*

low-fat foods are still part of the daily web of life tend to enjoy low blood pressure even as their hair turns gray.

In other words, say many experts, high blood pressure may not be an inevitable consequence of growing older. More likely, it's caused by the lifestyle habits many of us embrace in middle age—overeating, underexercising, and not getting enough fruits, vegetables, whole grains, and low-fat dairy products—that send the national blood pressure steadily upward.

Male or female?

Men under the age of 55 are more likely than women to have high blood pressure. But if you're a woman, don't let that news cause you to sit back and relax. Once women reach 55, their blood pressure tends to catch up and even surpass that of their male peers. In the past, experts often blamed menopause—or, more specifically, the drop in estrogen that accompanies menopause—for the tendency of older women to have higher blood pressure, but recent evidence has shown that estrogen actually has little effect on lowering blood pressure.

Family ties

Genetics cuts both ways. Sure, you might have inherited your mother's baby blues, but you might have also got stuck with your father's high blood pressure. The condition tends to run in

The Pill and Pressure

If you've just gone on the Pill or have been on it for awhile, listen up: You may experience a rise in blood pressure. You're most at risk of having this reaction to the Pill if you are overweight, have a family history of high blood pressure, or have kidney disease. (You should also know that taking the Pill and smoking are a particularly deadly duo, greatly increasing your risk for heart attack and stroke.)

Be sure to have your blood pressure checked before going on the Pill. Have it rechecked two to three months later and then once a year after that. If your blood pressure goes up while you're on the Pill, your doctor will either adjust the dosage or have you switch to some other form of contraception.

families. In fact, some evidence suggests that 30 to 60 percent of all cases of high blood pressure may be inherited. Having a parent with high blood pressure increases your risk for developing it yourself—but not as much, according to recent research, as having a brother or sister with coronary artery disease (also known as coronary arteriosclerosis).

What's responsible for high blood pressure's heirloom quality? Genes, of course. But the experts think lifestyle factors may also be at work. Families tend to share the same eating and exercise habits—and the same tendency to carry around excess body weight.

The racial element

In industrialized countries, certain racial and ethnic groups are more—or less—likely than others to develop high blood pressure. Here's what the statistics show for people living in the United States.

> If you are white, your risk of suffering from high blood pressure is about 25 percent.

> If you are Native American, your risk for HBP is only slightly higher.

> If you are Hispanic, it's slightly lower.

> If you are African American, your risk is through the roof—about 36 percent.

All of these numbers are too high, but the percentage of African Americans with high blood pressure is particularly alarming. Not only do more African Americans develop the condition, they also tend to do so at an early age. In addition, their high blood pressure is often more severe and progresses more rapidly. The bottom line is grim: High blood pressure accounts for 20 percent of all premature deaths among African Americans—twice the number for whites.

The Slave Trade Theory

Many scholars believe that slaves who had a genetic predisposition to retaining salt were more likely to survive the salt-wasting conditions of the brutal slave ship voyages from Africa to America of past centuries—conditions that often led to diarrhea, dehydration, and death. It makes sense then, say the scholars, that American descendants of the surviving slaves are also sensitive to salt—and more likely to develop high blood pressure.

That's the theory. But there are several problems with it. For example: Africans who have moved to Europe or North America in recent decades also have higher blood pressure than whites do. As a result of this and other evidence, most scientists today dismiss the slave trade theory and cite lifestyle and/or general genetic factors as the more likely reasons why high blood pressure is so common among African Americans.

Bad genes or Big Macs? Heredity is often cited as a reason for the statistical spike among African Americans, but experts say lifestyle choices—particularly being overweight, eating too many salty, fatty foods, and not exercising—are also contributing factors. Here's why: High blood pressure is very low among Africans; in fact, people living in rural West Africa have some of the lowest blood pressure levels in the world. Compare that with African Americans, who have some of the highest rates of high blood pressure in the world.

In addition, according to Dr. James Lynch of Johns Hopkins University Medical School, many African Americans are victims of environmental and socioeconomic stresses that might increase their risk for high blood pressure. His study showed that stress experienced by people living at low socioeconomic strata leads to poor self-image and high blood pressure. Combine this with the fact that these same people have poor access to health care and that might partially explain the higher correlation of African Americans and HBP.

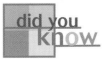

What's Your "Heartstyle"?

You know you have high blood pressure—or perhaps you know that you're at risk for developing it. Now that you've started reading this book, you also know that there are things you can do to get your BP under control. But here is the million-dollar question: Will you?

The answer may depend on your "heartstyle"—your particular attitude toward your high blood pressure and your overall health. According to a study conducted by Michael Weber, M.D., and his colleagues at the State University of New York, people who have been diagnosed with high blood pressure fit one of four distinct "heartstyle" profiles:

Actively Attentives. These can-do patients actively take charge of their high blood pressure. They modify their diet, increase their exercise, and do everything else their doctor requires to lower their risk factors. Weber's study found that 39 percent of people with high blood pressure fall into this group.

Nonchalant Newcomers. These patients, who represent 23 percent of the people diagnosed with high blood pressure, refuse to grasp the seriousness of their condition and therefore are less likely to do much to control it. They may take medication, but they usually do so only to keep their doctor happy.

> **Pressure Point:** Blood pressure tends to creep up during winter and slide back down during summer. Scientists think this seasonal fluctuation has more to do with changes in the length of the day rather than with changes in temperature.

Honestly Overwhelmed. Self-confidence is an issue for the 22 percent of high blood pressure patients who fall into this group. They tend to have lives that are beset with a host of problems, which lead them to feel helpless and to be negligent about taking proper care of themselves.

did you know

▶ *Eleven states in the southeastern United States have been dubbed the "Stroke Belt States" because the people living there are more likely to die from stroke than people living in other regions of the country. And guess what? Those same states (Alabama, Arkansas, Georgia, Indiana, Kentucky, Louisiana, Mississippi, North Carolina, South Carolina, Tennessee, and Virginia) also have a greater number of people with high blood pressure, which is one of the key risk factors for stroke.*

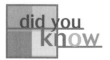

did you know

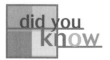

▶ *Blood pressure is just one of the pieces of physiological data (along with pulse, respiration, and sweat gland activity) that polygraphs, or lie-detector tests, use to determine whether or not a person is lying. According to advocates of these tests, your blood pressure changes ever so slightly when you're telling a fib. Of course, not everyone believes the tests are accurate, which is one of the reasons why accused criminals are not required to take them.*

Mainly Meds. Unwilling to alter their lifestyle, the 16 percent of patients with high blood pressure who fall into this group rely solely on medications to control their condition. They make no (or very, very little) effort to change their bad habits.

Which "heartstyle" is yours? Because you're reading this book, you are probably one of the Actively Attentives. You understand the seriousness of your condition and are highly motivated to make the crucial lifestyle changes necessary to get your blood pressure under control. Maybe you've already started taking better care of yourself and are reading this book only as a "refresher" course. Obviously, people who are "actively attentive" have the greatest chance of successfully lowering their blood pressure and getting their health back on track. But if you fall into one of the other groups, don't give up. Just reading this book may help empower you to take charge of your condition and to start making changes.

A Thoroughly Modern Malady

Until the twentieth century, few people died of heart disease. And nobody worried about high blood pressure or really even knew what it was. The condition grew in tandem with the flood of technological advances—such as automobiles, elevators, washing machines, and TV remotes. Technology was a double-edged blessing: It saved us the physical effort we needed to stay healthy.

Blood Pressure: As Time Goes By

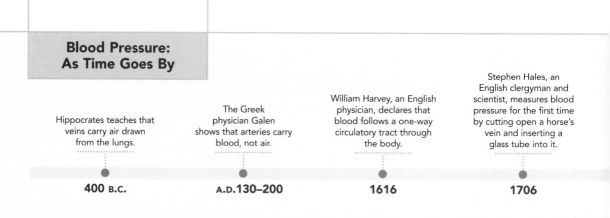

Hippocrates teaches that veins carry air drawn from the lungs.

The Greek physician Galen shows that arteries carry blood, not air.

William Harvey, an English physician, declares that blood follows a one-way circulatory tract through the body.

Stephen Hales, an English clergyman and scientist, measures blood pressure for the first time by cutting open a horse's vein and inserting a glass tube into it.

400 B.C.   **A.D. 130–200**   **1616**   **1706**

Machines also made it possible to mass-produce high-fat treats, such as ice cream and potato chips, which before had to be painstakingly prepared by hand in home kitchens. What's more, smoking took off in a big way during the twentieth century, especially with the free distribution of cigarettes to soldiers during both world wars.

These lifestyle changes led inevitably to damaged blood vessels, which in turn led to an increase in heart attacks and strokes. But, of course, putting together the cause (changing lifestyles) and effect (higher blood pressure, clogged arteries, and more heart disease) took some time—and a major scientific effort known as the Framingham Heart Study.

Tracking Down the Mystery Killer

After World War II, the United States emerged to find itself amid an epidemic of heart disease. A growing number of seemingly healthy people, especially men in their 50s and 60s, were suddenly keeling over dead from heart attacks. No one knew why. (Remember: This was in the dark days before preventive medicine. Scientists weren't even sure if cigarettes caused cancer.)

The study that started it all. In 1948, the federal government, under the auspices of the National Heart Institute (now known as the National Heart, Lung, and Blood Institute), decided to launch a study to see if there was some hidden link between the way people lived and the fate of their hearts. Scientists descended upon the town of Framingham, Massachusetts, where they persuaded about 5,000 healthy residents (roughly one-fifth of the town's total population) to submit to a physical exam every two years for the next 20 years.

Rene T. H. Laennec, a French physician, invents the stethoscope.

The Czechoslovakian-born physician Samuel von Basch invents the first practical sphygmomanometer for estimating blood pressure.

Italian physician and inventor Scipione Riva-Rocci introduces a new, easier-to-use, and more accurate sphygmomanometer.

American surgeon Harvey Cushing demonstrates the value of observing blood pressure during medical operations.

1816　　　**1880**　　　**1896**　　　**1900**

then and now

▶ *Although the medical community today sees diet as an indispensable part of lowering blood pressure, back in the 1930s and '40s, doctors ignored—or ridiculed—efforts like those of Duke University's Walter Kempner, who as early as 1939 was advising patients to change their diets to lower their blood pressure. Kempner's recommended diet, which consisted mostly of rice and fruit, seemed particularly bizarre in those meat-and-potatoes days of American cuisine.*

> **Pressure Point:** Although it seems as if we've heard about "risk factors" forever, the term was actually first coined in a 1961 research paper from the Framingham Heart Study.

Thus began one of the longest and most influential medical studies in history. In the ensuing 50-plus years (the study has been extended to include later generations of Framingham residents), scientists have used data from the Framingham study to publish more than 1,000 research papers. These reports, like the one in 1964 that finally fingered cigarette smoking as a menace to the heart, have changed—and saved—the lives of millions of people.

The landmark study certainly turned opinions about high blood pressure on their head. Before the study began, doctors thought the condition was a necessary part of getting older. In fact, they thought older people needed high blood pressure to push blood through their narrower arteries and prevent stroke. As a result, many doctors were horrified when medications to help patients lower their blood pressure became available during the 1950s. Use of such medications, they thought, constituted malpractice when, in truth, the drugs could have saved countless lives by lowering blood pressure to safe levels.

Unmasking a killer. But by 1971, even the most recalcitrant doctors saw the light. That was the year Framingham research revealed high blood pressure to be a bad thing at any age. The data clearly showed that the higher blood pressure climbed, the

---

Russian physician Dr. Nicolai Korotkoff uses a blood pressure cuff and a stethoscope to show the relationship between the pulse and the contracting and resting phases of the heart.

Walter Kempner of Duke University theorizes that blood pressure can be lowered through diet.

Chronic high blood pressure kills President Franklin Delano Roosevelt.

The National Heart Institute launches the Framingham Heart Study to see whether lifestyle choices contribute to heart disease.

1905   **1939**   **1945**   **1948**

greater the risk for heart disease and stroke. By this time Framingham had also revealed, much to many doctors' chagrin, a strong, indisputable link between high blood pressure and such lifestyle factors as diet, weight, smoking, and exercise (or the lack thereof).

High Blood Pressure: Public Enemy No. 1

People are much more aware of high blood pressure today than they were several decades ago—thanks in large part to the tireless efforts of the National High Blood Pressure

Roosevelt's Reckoning

The medical records of Franklin D. Roosevelt, thirty-second president of the United States, show that his blood pressure more than doubled to severely high levels during the last 10 years of his life. Doctors did not treat his steadily climbing blood pressure because it was considered unwise to do so at the time. Yet even if White House doctors had wanted to lower the president's blood pressure, they didn't have the medications back then to do it.

According to Roosevelt's personal physician, the stroke that killed the president on April 12, 1945, "came out of the clear blue sky." It would take years before scientists would clearly connect high blood pressure to stroke and before doctors would begin treating the condition aggressively.

Medications for high blood pressure become available.

The Framingham Heart Study shows high blood pressure to be a risk factor for heart disease and stroke.

The DASH Study shows that diet can lower blood pressure.

The DASH II Study shows that eating less sodium significantly lowers blood pressure.

1950   **1971**   **1997**   **2001**

Education Program, a public-awareness campaign run by a variety of professional and voluntary groups and coordinated by the National Heart, Lung, and Blood Institute of the National Institutes of Health.

In 1972, before the education program started, less than 25 percent of people in the United States knew that high blood pressure could lead to stroke and heart attack. Today, 68 percent of Americans are aware of that deadly fact. Also, many more people are controlling their high blood pressure today—27 percent compared with a dismal 10 percent back in the 1970s.

> **Pressure Point:** Researchers believe that hypertension medications have saved the lives of more than 1 million people since 1980 alone.

No question about it: The National High Blood Pressure Education Program has saved lives. Deaths from strokes have plummeted 60 percent and deaths from coronary artery disease have fallen nearly 53 percent in the United States during the past three decades.

But no one's declaring victory yet—not by a long shot. First, the fact that 27 percent of Americans have their high blood pressure under control means that 73 percent don't. And second, recent trends haven't been as encouraging as the earlier ones. For example:

> Improvements in high blood pressure awareness and control have slowed and even slightly declined since 1993. (For evidence of this backsliding trend, see *Your Wake-Up Call*, right.)

> The percentage of people having strokes has risen slightly during the past decade.

> The rate of decline in coronary artery disease appears to be leveling off.

> Doctors are seeing an increase in new cases of kidney failure that require dialysis (a procedure that uses a machine to perform kidneylike functions, such as filtering blood and

Your Wake-Up Call

Americans need to "wake up" to the dangers of high blood pressure. That's what researchers from the Mayo Clinic declared in a troubling 1999 study. After examining 630 randomly chosen Minnesotans for high blood pressure, the researchers asked the subjects two questions: 1) Has a doctor ever told you that you had high blood pressure? and 2) Are you currently taking any medications for blood pressure?

Now the troubling part: The researchers found that 370 of the people examined had high blood pressure, but less than 40 percent knew it. And of the 44 percent of the study's subjects with high blood pressure who were being treated for the condition, only about 17 percent had it under control. A similar study conducted within the same community more than a decade earlier had shown more promising results. Do you hear the distant sound of an alarm going off?

ridding the body of harmful wastes, extra salt, and fluids). Diabetics need dialysis more than any other patient suffering from a condition; people with high blood pressure are second.

Despite these setbacks, however, the national offensive against high blood pressure has experienced remarkable success. The fact that you're reading this book is a measure of that success. It shows you're among the 68 percent who are at least aware of high blood pressure's serious health risks. Now, of course, it's time to become one of the 27 percent who are actually doing something about lowering those risks. Just remember: You are the architect of your own blood pressure. Only you can limit your salt and alcohol intake, stop smoking, and make sure you get enough exercise.

It's time to take charge of your high blood pressure!

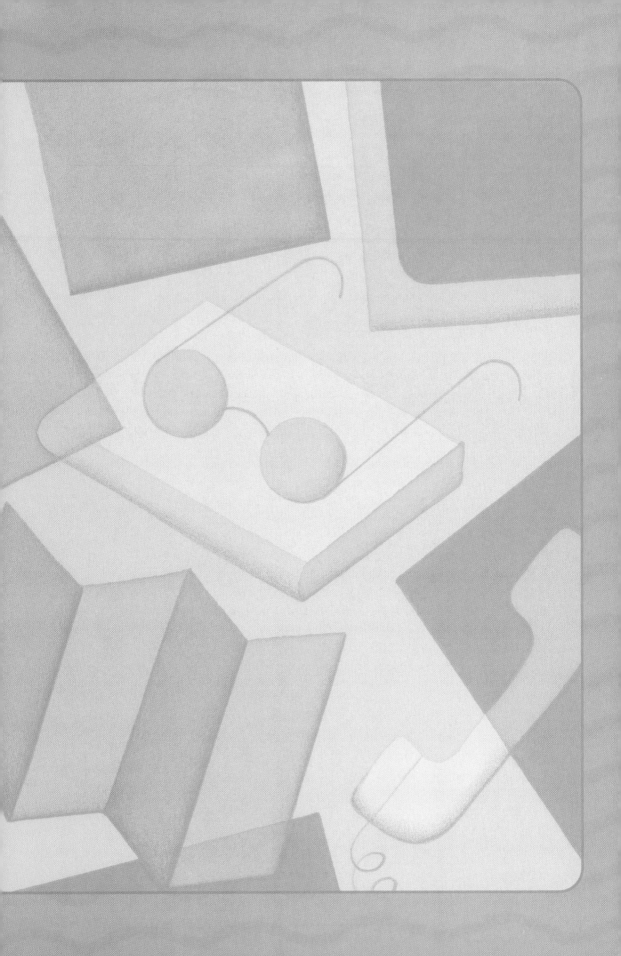

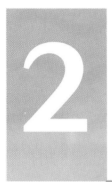

The Lowdown on High Blood Pressure

As one old rock song concludes, "It all comes

down to you." Ditto for high blood pressure.

The good news is that there is a lot you can

do to keep it in check. Knowing about high

blood pressure's devastating effects on your

vital organs can often turn a passive person

into a proactive advocate for lowering it.

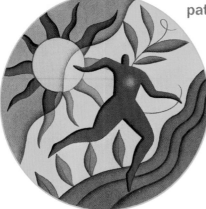

KEY CONCEPT Studies show that an underinformed patient is an undertreated patient. Learning as much as you can about high blood pressure can help you overcome it.

Knowledge Is Power

Before you can understand what high blood pressure is, you need to know how blood pressure works. And to understand that, you need to know something about your cardiovascular system, which consists of your heart (the cardio part) and the huge, intricate web of blood vessels (the vascular part) that weaves its way through every inch of tissue in your body.

Sound too technical or boring? Are you thinking maybe of fast forwarding to the chapters on treatment? You'd be wise not to. The more you understand about the miraculous workings of your heart and blood vessels, the better you'll be able to grasp why it's so important—indeed, crucial—to keep your blood pressure under control.

Take it seriously. Studies conducted by the National Heart, Lung, and Blood Institute found that only *after* gaining a thorough understanding of the consequences and prognosis of untreated high blood pressure are people persuaded to regard the condition with the seriousness it deserves. This chapter will also enlighten you about how the action steps outlined in Chapter 1 fit into the picture—and how following them may literally save your life.

A Pressure Primer

Your heart has the starring role in the blood pressure story, beating an average of 70 times a minute. With each beat, it releases a rush of blood from its left ventricle, or main pumping chamber (see illustration on page 39). The blood exits the left ventricle through the aorta, the body's largest blood vessel, and quickly spreads throughout your body via an amazingly complex network of blood vessels. In fact, if laid end-to-end, your body's blood vessels would stretch more than 60,000 miles, or twice around the Earth's equator!

The force is with you. One of your heart's main jobs is to create pressure in your aorta so that the oxygen- and nutrient-rich blood that leaves the heart will be pushed throughout your body to your cells—all 100 trillion of them. The aorta branches off into smaller arteries and then into even smaller and thinner ones, known as arterioles. Simply put, blood pressure is the force of blood flowing through your arteries and pushing against their vessel walls.

> **Pressure Point:** It takes only one minute for your heart to pump all of your blood supply—about 5 quarts —through your body. Each day, therefore, your heart pumps more than 2,000 gallons of blood.

The smallest blood vessels in your body are the capillaries, which swap oxygen and nutrients from the arterioles for carbon dioxide and other waste products from your cells. Once that switch has taken place, the heart's pressure on the blood enables the "spent" blood to travel back to the heart through a different system of blood vessels known as the veins. Like a train or bus making all local stops, the blood first stops off at the lungs, where it gets a refill of oxygen. Then it goes on to the heart, where it is pumped back out into the aorta and starts the journey all over again.

So some pressure in your blood vessels is a good—even vital—thing.

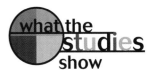

what the studies show

▶ *According to new data from the Hypertension Optimal Treatment (HOT) study, people over age 65 with high blood pressure respond better than younger people to hypertension treatment. Older patients treated with a calcium antagonist (an HBP drug) achieved lower blood pressure levels, were less likely to experience side effects, and needed fewer medications to reach their blood pressure targets than younger patients.*

BP: Plumbing Its Inner Workings

To better understand how blood pressure works, picture your kitchen faucet. A large city pump (think heart) sends water (think blood) from an underground reservoir or other source into the pipes (think arteries) in your home. When you turn on the faucet, pressure pushes the water into your sink (think cells). The water then runs down the drain and into more pipes (think veins), which takes it back to a water processing plant to be cleaned and recycled.

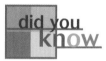

did you know

▶ *Blood shoots out of the heart's aorta, or largest blood vessel, at the phenomenal rate of 15 inches per second. By the time it reaches the tiny capillaries in your fingers and toes, however, the flow of blood has slowed down considerably to a rate of 0.02 inches per second.*

Normal Ups and Downs

Your blood pressure is literally on a roller-coaster ride throughout the day. In general, it goes up when you're active and goes down when you're resting. Your BP is usually the lowest during sleep because your bodily processes downshift, creating less demand for oxygen. On the other hand, when you're working your body hard—whether it be running to catch a bus or lifting weights at the gym—your muscles cry out for more oxygen. Your heart then responds by pumping out more blood, which elevates your blood pressure.

Even when you stand up—say, after sitting at your desk or in a movie theater—your blood pressure shoots up a bit. Your brain recognizes that blood has collected in your legs while you were sitting, so it jacks up your blood pressure to get that blood back into circulation.

➤ **Pressure Point:** High blood pressure is not a reflection of your personality. Many calm, relaxed, even-tempered people get high blood pressure; many tense and uptight people have perfectly normal blood pressure.

Many other factors can also raise your blood pressure temporarily, including eating (your body needs extra blood for digestion), drinking alcohol, stress, and strong emotions like fear and anger. Your blood pressure also fluctuates according to the time of day: It tends to be highest in the morning just after you've awakened (a time when your brain needs more blood and oxygen) and lowest in the evening (when your brain is ratcheting down).

All these daily ups and downs are normal and don't typically cause a problem. You usually need to worry only when your blood pressure slowly climbs above a healthy level and stays there month after month, year after year.

The Goldilocks Syndrome

You don't want your blood pressure to go too high or too low. You want it to be within a normal, healthy range—or, as fabled Goldilocks put it, "just right." Fortunately, your body is constantly trying to adjust your blood pressure to that "just right" level. It accomplishes it using three main tools: your heart, arteries, and kidneys.

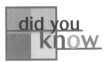

did you know

▶ If you work the night shift, your blood pressure rises when you rise, not when the sun does. That's because your body has shifted its daily, or circadian, rhythms—including that of your blood pressure—to match your new sleep/wake cycle.

How Your Heart Works

Your heartbeat consists of two stages: **Systole (left),** in which your heart muscle forces blood out of the pumping chamber (ventricles). Blood on the right side of the heart goes to your lungs and that on the left side is pumped into the aorta that feeds your arteries. During **diastole (right),** your heart muscle relaxes and expands to allow blood to flow into the pumping chambers from your holding chambers (**atria**).

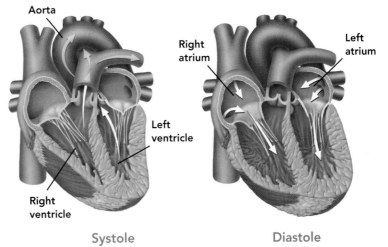

Systole

Diastole

Your heart

As we've already said, the pumping action of your heart raises and lowers your blood pressure. The harder your heart has to work (when you're shoveling snow, for example, or when you're tensed up during a job interview), the greater the pressure on your arteries. The opposite is also true: When you're calm and relaxed (say, lounging on a peaceful tropical beach), your heart pumps slower, lessening the pressure on your blood vessels.

Your arteries

The width of your arteries also affects your blood pressure. To accommodate the surge of blood coming from your heart, your arteries are lined with smooth muscles that can expand or contract as blood flows through them. The more wide open and "elastic" your arteries are, the less resistant they are to the flow of blood and the less force that's exerted on their walls. The less elastic your arteries, the harder your heart has to work to push blood through them.

Your kidneys

These are the "forgotten" blood-pressure regulators, the ones most people don't know about. But your kidneys do play a big role in your blood pressure's ups and downs. They control how much sodium your body contains and thus how much water stays in your blood. (Sodium retains water.) More water means more blood trying to cram its way through blood vessels, and that means more pressure on the walls of those vessels. Less water, of course, means less blood and lower pressure.

Your brain weighs in

Your heart, arteries, and kidneys may be the major players in regulating your blood pressure, but they are by no means the only ones. Your brain and a complex system of hormones and enzymes are also intimately involved in the process.

Spies for the brain. The brain enters the picture through the aid of tiny nerve endings called baroreceptors, nodes or sensors that hide out in the walls of major arteries as well as in the heart and lungs. The baroreceptors act like spies, monitoring the pressure of blood. Whenever they sense a change, they quickly send a message to the brain, which issues orders for the body to release an artillery of hormones to get the heart to

Atherosclerosis

Atherosclerosis—the clogging of arteries with fatty deposits—can elevate your blood pressure. Here's how it works: Plaque deposits gradually accumulate in the lining of your arteries. As the deposits enlarge, blood circulation decreases and blood pressure increases. This elevates your risk for heart attack, stroke, and other vascular problems.

Normal artery

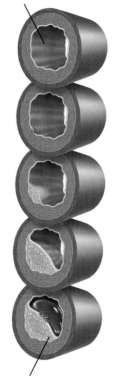

Atherosclerotic artery

either slow down or speed up and the arteries to either widen or narrow.

Two of the hormones that get their original marching orders from the brain are epinephrine and norepinephrine, also known as adrenaline and noradrenaline. When you're highly stressed or tense, such as when a sudden noise frightens you or when you're doing public speaking, the brain signals the adrenal glands to release these hormones—known, not surprisingly, as "stress hormones"—which surge through your body. They cause your heart to pump more rapidly and your arteries to narrow, which then raises your blood pressure.

A terrible trio. Three other hormones—renin, angiotensin, and aldosterone—also team up to regulate blood pressure. The process starts with the enzyme renin, produced mainly by cells in the kidneys. Once released into the blood, renin searches out and eventually reacts with the protein angiotensin (made by the liver) to form a new and much more powerful compound, angiotensin II.

Raising blood pressure is one of angiotensin II's key jobs and it performs this task in two ways: First, it orders blood vessels to narrow. Second, it helps create aldosterone, a hormone that causes the kidneys to stock up on sodium (salt). Remember: The more sodium in the body, the more fluid is retained—and the more fluid, the higher the blood pressure.

Some medications—ACE (angiotensin-converting enzyme) inhibitors and angiotensin II receptor blockers—lower blood pressure by controlling this trio of hormones.

Saying NO to High Blood Pressure

In recent years, scientists have added nitric oxide, a molecule in the body, to the known arsenal of blood-pressure regulators. Made from an amino acid called L-arginine, nitric oxide has been found to relax and open blood vessels—and that, of course, helps lower blood pressure.

Some people, however, are unable to convert L-arginine into nitric oxide. That's not good, because it means their blood vessels remain tight and stiff—and their blood pressure climbs. Scientists haven't a clue (yet) why the conversion fails to take place.

The Hard Truth About High Blood Pressure

Perpetual high blood pressure is hard on your body. Real hard. Your major organs—especially your arteries, heart, brain, kidneys, and eyes—aren't equipped to handle constant pressure. They need time to relax and recuperate—or they suffer the consequences.

The medical evidence is clear: If untreated, high blood pressure can wreak havoc on your body, causing serious medical problems. Here's how, over time, your various organs succumb to the pressure.

Your Blood Pressure Goes Up When...

...Your heart pumps with more force
...Your blood vessels narrow
...Your blood vessels lose their flexibility and become hard and stiff
...Your blood volume increases

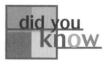

did you know

▶ *Blood pressure is strongest in the aorta, the artery that leads out of the left ventricle of the heart. How strong? If the aorta should get cut, blood would squirt out five or six feet!*

How Pressure Gets to Your Arteries

Uncontrolled high blood pressure can put in motion a vicious cycle of events that makes it increasingly more difficult for your arteries to move blood through your body—a potentially dangerous development known as atherosclerosis.

The strait and narrow. The cycle goes like this: The constant pressure of extra blood pounding through your arteries thickens and hardens the arterial muscles, narrowing the blood vessels' passageway. The elevated pressure also damages the arteries' inner lining. Blood cells (called monocytes and platelets) and fat deposits gather at the damaged areas, forming a hard plaque that further narrows the channel through which blood can flow. (Picture rust collecting on the inside of metal pipes.)

Coming to Terms

Hardening of the arteries is known as arteriosclerosis, from the Greek word *sklerosis,* which means "hardening." The clogging of the arteries with fatty deposits and platelets is known as atherosclerosis, from the Greek word *ather,* which means "porridge." (Scientists long ago thought the soft fat deposits resembled their breakfast fare.) These two terms, however, are often used interchangeably. In *Taking Charge of High Blood Pressure*, we follow the popular practice of referring to them both as atherosclerosis.

This is very bad news for your organs and tissues, whose blood supply is greatly diminished by the process. It's especially hard on your heart, which has to pump more vigorously to force the blood through your narrowed arteries. The harder your heart pumps, the greater your blood pressure—and the more damage to your arteries. And so it goes.

One more problem. When a blood vessel weakens, its wall may form a saclike bulge known as an aneurysm. Eventually, the aneurysm may leak or burst, flooding surrounding tissue in blood—a life-threatening event. Aneurysms are most likely to develop in a brain artery or in your aorta, especially where the artery passes through your abdomen.

Watch Out! Signs of an Aneurysm

Unfortunately, aneurysms seldom produce any symptoms in their early stages. Advanced aneurysms, however, do sometimes send out warning signs. If you experience any of the following symptoms, call your doctor right away:

- Severe headache that doesn't go away
- Constant abdominal or back pain
- Dizziness
- Nosebleeds
- Blurred vision

How Pressure Gets to Your Heart

High blood pressure is double trouble for your heart. First, it raises your risk for developing coronary artery disease, or damage to the major blood vessels (the coronary arteries) that feed your heart. Plaque is the culprit, of course. The buildup of plaque narrows the coronary arteries, reducing the amount of blood that flows through them.

Eventually, your heart muscle can't get enough oxygen to meet your body's demands on it. Any effort, whether it be walking briskly, doing yard work, or even having sex, puts added strain on your heart and may trigger angina, a temporary pain in the chest. Angina is really your heart's attempt to get your attention. You should heed the warning and seek treatment. If you don't, the flow of blood to your heart may eventually stop altogether, and you'll suffer a heart attack.

> **Pressure Point:** People with high blood pressure are more likely to die from coronary artery disease and its complications—such as a heart attack—than from any other cause.

Job burnout. High blood pressure can also wear out your heart. The higher your blood pressure, the harder your heart muscle is working to pump blood into your aorta. Like any other muscle in your body, the extra workout causes your heart to get bigger, especially the walls of its main pumping chamber, the left ventricle. This enlargement is known as left ventricular hypertrophy. But, in this case, bigger isn't better. The thickening of the left ventricle's walls reduces the amount of blood that the chamber can hold, which forces the heart to pump harder to keep enough blood moving through the body. As a result, the heart enlarges and weakens even more.

Where does it all end? Often, sadly, with congestive heart failure, a condition in which the enlarged and worn-out heart simply can't pump fast enough to keep blood circulating adequately. Fluid from backed-up blood in the vessels seeps into small airways in the lungs, making them "congested" and causing shortness of breath. Fluid may also collect in the legs and ankles, a swelling condition known as edema. Eventually—if the condition isn't treated—the heart simply gives up and stops pumping altogether.

Watch Out! Signs of Heart Attack

If you experience any of the following symptoms, seek emergency medical care immediately:

- ◗ Uncomfortable tightness or pain in your chest
- ◗ Pain that extends from the chest to the shoulders, arms (especially the left arm), or neck
- ◗ Dizziness, fainting, sweating, nausea, or shortness of breath

How Pressure Gets to Your Brain

Possibility 1: High blood pressure helps create the buildup of plaque that narrows an artery feeding the brain. A blood clot gets stuck in the constricted space, blocking the flow of blood. Starved of oxygen, brain cells quickly start to die. This is known as an ischemic stroke and can be fatal.

Possibility 2: The pressure weakens the walls of a brain artery leading to a balloonlike bulge called an aneurysm. When the aneurysm bursts, blood spills into the brain, building up pressure under the skull and damaging surrounding tissue. This is a hemorrhagic stroke, and it, too, can be fatal.

Possibility 3: A clot blocks the flow of blood to the brain, but not completely or only for a very short time. Some brain cells are permanently damaged, but usually in small, unnoticeable ways—at first, that is. Research now suggests that over time these "mini-strokes" (officially known as transient ischemic attacks, or TIAs) can slow down a person's thinking skills and increase the risk for developing dementia. TIAs are

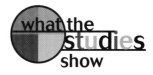

what the **studies** show

◗ *If you control your blood pressure for five years or more, your risk of having a heart attack will drop by 20 percent. Even better news: Your risk of having congestive heart failure will be cut in half.*

◗ *According to a study in the* Archives of Internal Medicine, *pulse pressure may be an accurate predictor of cardiovascular complications in older people with high blood pressure. Pulse pressure reflects the stiffness of arteries, which may be just as important in determining heart attack risk as blocked arteries.*

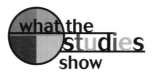

▶ Researchers at the National Institutes of Health found that people with high blood pressure—but who were otherwise healthy— had poorer memory and slower thinking skills than people of the same age who didn't have high blood pressure. Now for the good news: Another study showed that this brain drain can be avoided if you vigorously work to maintain lower blood pressure. The researchers theorized that treating high blood pressure prevents blood vessels from hardening, thus ensuring a healthy flow of blood to the brain.

also strong warning signs that you may be at increased risk for a full-fledged ischemic stroke.

Watch Out! Signs of a Stroke

If you experience any of the following symptoms, seek emergency medical care immediately:

- ◖ Sudden numbness or weakness of the face, arm, or leg, especially on one side of the body
- ◖ Sudden mental confusion
- ◖ Sudden difficulty with speaking or understanding speech
- ◖ Sudden trouble seeing in one or both eyes
- ◖ Sudden trouble walking, dizziness, loss of balance or coordination
- ◖ Sudden, severe headache with no known cause

How Pressure Gets to Your Kidneys

High blood pressure can interfere with one of your kidneys' all-important duties: filtering out waste products in your blood so the waste can be excreted in your urine. High blood pressure throws a wrench in this process by either narrowing the arteries that lead into your kidneys or by directly damaging the ones within them (or by doing both).

> **Pressure Point:** High blood pressure is responsible for 25 percent of all kidney failures. Only diabetes causes more kidneys to stop functioning.

Either way, without a generous supply of blood, your kidneys become less efficient, making it doubly tough on the organs. Your kidneys are already less efficient at removing fluid due to the damage caused by high blood pressure. This, in turn, can lead to even higher blood pressure, since your kidneys won't be able to remove excess fluid and sodium from the bloodstream, which further damages the organs.

Stopping the madness. Unless the cycle is stopped, your

kidneys eventually throw in the towel and shut down altogether. This is known as end-stage renal disease. When you reach it, you'll need either dialysis treatment to maintain kidney function (and to keep yourself alive) or a transplant operation for a brand-new kidney.

Watch Out! Signs of Kidney Disease

If you experience any of these symptoms, call your doctor:

- Frequent need to urinate, especially at night
- Difficulty urinating
- Pain or burning when you urinate
- Puffiness around your eyes and swelling of your hands and feet
- Pain in your lower back
- Unpleasant taste and odor in your mouth

How Pressure Gets to Your Eyes

It's the same old story: High blood pressure threatens your vision by damaging your arteries, although this time the victims are the delicate vessels that supply blood to your eyes. Your eye doctor can actually see this damage when he or she examines your peepers. In fact, atherosclerosis—and high blood pressure—are often diagnosed during an eye exam. If the blood vessels in your eyes are damaged, there's a good chance blood vessels elsewhere in your body are also under pressure. And wherever atherosclerosis can be found, high blood pressure is likely lurking, too.

When the eyes have it. The part of your eye most susceptible to high blood pressure damage is the retina, the nerve layer at the back of the eye that senses light and sends visual images back to your brain. Weakened arteries in the retina can burst, leaking blood and fluid into surrounding tissue. This is a serious complication that can result in lost vision.

If you've been diagnosed with high blood pressure, you should make a point of seeing an eye doctor (ophthalmologist) at least once a year. Fortunately, when you lower your high blood pressure, you also lower your risk for developing serious eye problems. But even after you've gotten

did you know

The vast majority of strokes—some 70 percent—are caused by high blood pressure. By lowering your high blood pressure, you reduce your risk of having a stroke sevenfold.

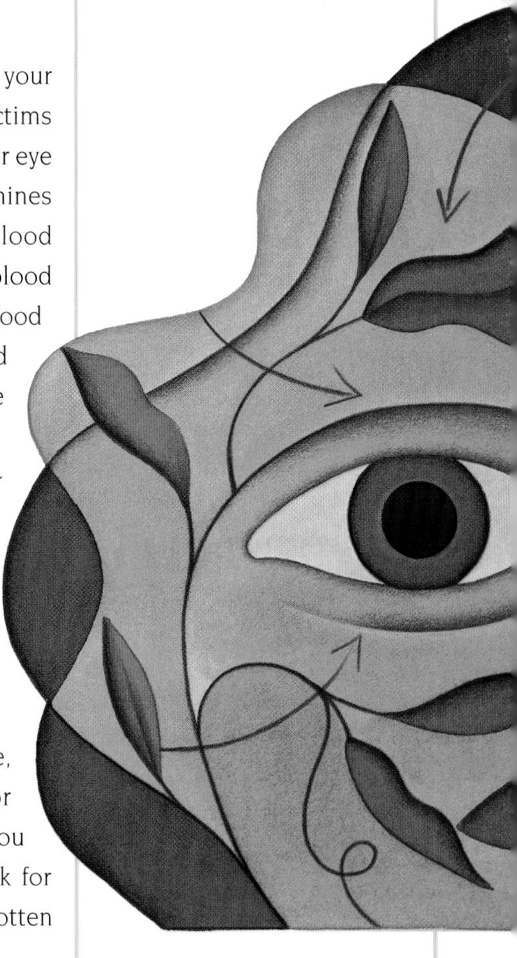

your blood pressure under control, you should continue, as a precautionary measure, to have your eyes examined annually.

> **Watch Out! Signs of Vision Problems**
>
> If you experience any of the following symptoms, call your doctor immediately:
>
> ○ You see "flashes" of light or tiny objects floating in your eyes
>
> ○ You notice a "veil" or "shadow" over part of your vision
>
> ○ Your vision becomes blurred or hazy

The Two Faces of High Blood Pressure

If you suffer from HBP, you have either primary (essential) or secondary high blood pressure. The odds are that you have primary HBP. In fact, 95 percent of people diagnosed with the condition have this type.

The Essential Difference

First, let's get down to terms: The old designation—essential high blood pressure—is really a misnomer. The term was coined in the early 1800s, and it seemed to fit until about 30 years ago, when scientists learned that having high blood pressure definitely wasn't essential to the aging process. (At one time, doctors had mistakenly thought that the higher your blood pressure, the better your chances of getting blood to your vital organs. The rule was that your blood pressure should be 100 plus your age.) In fact, we now know the only thing that is essential is treating and lowering high blood pressure. As a result, doctors today prefer to call this type of blood pressure primary rather than essential.

A condition in search of a cause. Primary high blood pressure has no obvious cause. That's why your doctor will probably shrug his or her shoulders when you ask, "Why me?"

> **Pressure Point:** Despite the fact that there are known risk factors for primary hypertension, researchers don't know why these factors lead to sustained, abnormal elevation of blood pressure.

Factors like diet, lack of exercise, excess weight, too much imbibing of alcohol, and smoking increase your risk. Various researchers have concluded that HBP risk factors are additive; the more you have, the better the chance you'll develop severe hypertension. The mystery to the medical community is that not everyone with the same risk factors develops high blood pressure, so something else must be going on.

Researchers are studying several genetic defects that might contribute to high blood pressure. Most experts, however, believe that primary high blood pressure is probably the result of the complex interaction of many factors—not all having to do with DNA. And different factors may affect different people, which perhaps explains why primary high blood pressure has no one-size-fits-all treatment. The good news is that most risk factors for primary high blood pressure can be controlled.

The Other HBP

Unlike primary hypertension, whose origins are mysterious and which can't be cured, secondary hypertension is caused by identifiable and, in many cases, correctable problems somewhere else in your body. If you have secondary HBP, you're in the minority: Only about 5 percent of people with high blood pressure have this type. Once the underlying cause of secondary high blood pressure is treated or cured, the pressure usually drops back down to normal. These problems include:

Kidney trouble. When there's a disease in the kidneys—inflammation or an injury, say—these filtering factories can't work to remove waste and excess water from the bloodstream. When kidneys realize that they are falling down on the job and not getting enough blood to accomplish their tasks, they send more of the hormone renin into the bloodstream to help raise

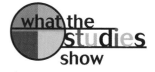

what the studies show

▶ *According to a study in* the Journal of the American Medical Association, *sleep apnea—an intermittent cessation of breathing during sleep—seems to be an independent risk factor for high blood pressure. Although researchers can't explain how sleep apnea increases risk, they encourage people who experience it to treat it either by losing weight or using a continuous positive airway pressure device that keeps airways open during sleep.*

blood pressure. As you would guess, the higher blood pressure isn't good for the rest of the body or the kidneys.

Aorta trouble. In this scenario, the aorta—the largest artery in the body—narrows abruptly at some point in the chest. As a result, your hard-working heart pumps even more vigorously to shuttle blood through the smaller opening. This elevates blood pressure above the narrowed part of the aorta while BP below the narrowed opening is normal or even low.

Pregnant Pause: HBP and Motherhood

If you have high blood pressure, you can have a normal pregnancy and a healthy baby. Millions of women with high blood pressure can testify to that. But having high blood pressure puts both you and your baby at greater risk for complications. Serious ones. You could experience seizures or kidney damage, for example. Your baby could be born prematurely or with brain damage. Such problems are rare but real.

It's best to talk with your doctor before you become pregnant. Some high blood pressure medications shouldn't be taken during pregnancy, so your doctor could very well want to change your prescription.

If you develop high blood pressure for the first time when you become pregnant—usually during the last three months of pregnancy—know that such pressure spikes tend to be mild and usually go back down once the pregnancy is over. Consider this episode a warning sign, however, that you are at risk for developing high blood pressure later in life.

Although medication is not necessary for mild cases of pregnancy-induced high blood pressure, your doctor may ask you to change your eating habits to include more whole grains, fruits, veggies, and low-fat dairy products—the kinds of foods that can help lower blood pressure.

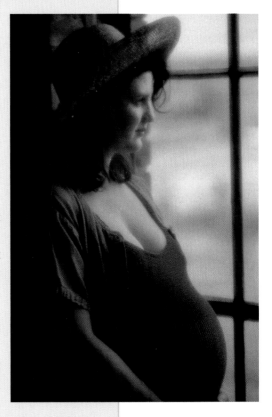

>**Pressure Point:** Hypertension in young children—a relatively uncommon phenomenon—is often due to a narrowed aorta. Over time, a child's aorta may grow large enough to work properly—or surgery can correct the problem.

Adrenal trouble. Located atop the kidneys, your adrenal glands release hormones that control everything from sexual function to food digestion. A tumor that develops on one of the glands can cause a variety of changes in the body, including increased blood pressure. Depending on where the tumor is located, it can cause the adrenal gland to produce too much of the hormones aldosterone, adrenaline, or cortisol—all of which can elevate blood pressure.

Thyroid trouble. Hormones made by your thyroid gland regulate all aspects of your metabolism. When the organ releases too much of a hormone, it could speed up your heart and overtax your cardiovascular system, leading to high blood pressure. A decrease in thyroid hormones can also increase high blood pressure for different reasons.

Medication trouble. You need to be on high alert when taking some medications. Although birth control pills increase most women's blood pressure only slightly, in a few cases, they can trigger the development of high blood pressure. Such

did you know

> *About one-quarter of women with pregnancy-induced high blood pressure develop a very serious condition called preeclampsia, usually quite suddenly. The three major signs of preeclampsia are a big rise in blood pressure, excessive swelling of the hands and feet, and a high level of protein in the urine (only a lab test can show this). Other symptoms include headaches, vision problems, and stomach pain. If you experience any of these symptoms during your pregnancy, call your doctor immediately.*

Secondary High Blood Pressure: The Tipoffs

- Did your high blood pressure come on suddenly?

- Do you have very high blood pressure readings?

- Do you have wide swings in blood pressure?

- Do you have other unusual symptoms?

If you answered yes to any of these questions, you may have secondary rather than primary high blood pressure. Talk with your doctor.

over-the-counter drugs as cold remedies, nasal decongestants, appetite suppressants, and nonsteroidal anti-inflammatory drugs (NSAIDs) can spike blood pressure (aspirin, however, doesn't have this effect), as can several prescription drugs, including cortisone and prednisone. Drinking heavily (three or more alcoholic drinks daily) or using illegal drugs, such as cocaine and amphetamines, can also elevate your BP.

Testing, Testing: Diagnosing HBP

Because blood pressure often doesn't cause symptoms until it's too late, you need to get it checked. Blood pressure checks require no needles, no drawing of blood, no invasive procedures. All you need to do is sit down for a few minutes, stick out your arm, and have a nurse or doctor perform a simple, painless test.

It's a Wrap

The device that measures blood pressure may be simple to use, but it is a mouthful to pronounce: Can you say sphygmomanometer (SFIG-mo-mah-NOM-uh-tur)? The first practical model was invented in 1880, and its design has been steadily improved upon since. The sphygmomanometer consists of an

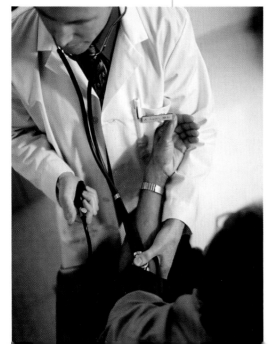

inflatable cuff, an air pump, and a gauge that often looks like a large thermometer. Some modern sphygmomanometers have a round dial activated by a spring-pressure gauge or are electronic and produce digital readouts. Each type of blood pressure gauge has its advantages and disadvantages (see right).

Here's how the device works: A rubber cuff is wrapped around your upper arm. The cuff is inflated with air, gradually compressing a large artery in the arm until the blood flow in that artery stops. Then a valve is opened to release air from the cuff, which allows blood to reflow in the artery.

Gauging the Gauges: Pros and Cons

If you decide to take your blood pressure at home—or your doctor recommends you do so—you have three good choices of sphygmomanometers. Most experts recommend the aneroid model.

Mercury

Advantages	Disadvantages
Durable; easy to read; needs no readjustment to stay accurate.	Sometimes unwieldy to carry; if broken, mercury can be hazardous; can be difficult to use for people who have trouble using their hands or those who have hearing problems.

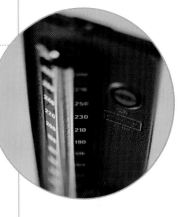

Spring-Gauge (aneroid)

Advantages	Disadvantages
Lightweight; portable; often inexpensive; some have extra-large dials for easier reading; some have built-in stethoscopes.	Must monitor accuracy of gauge annually by checking it against a mercury model; parts easily damaged; can be difficult to use for people who have trouble using their hands or those who have hearing problems.

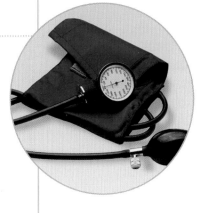

Electronic (digital)

Advantages	Disadvantages
Single unit makes it easy to use; portable; large, easy-to-read digital display; good for people who have trouble using their hands or those who have hearing problems.	Expensive; less accurate than mercury and spring-gauge models; must monitor accuracy of gauge by checking it annually against mercury model; parts easily damaged; sometimes produces inaccurate readings.

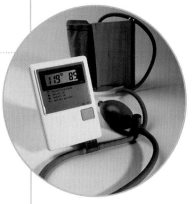

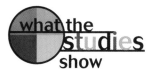

◗ *Before you phone home, consider this: German researchers have found that using a mobile phone for half an hour can significantly raise blood pressure. You don't have to be having a heated conversation—or any conversation, for that matter—for your blood pressure to rise. The radio-frequency electromagnetic fields (EMFs) emitted by mobile phones will perform that feat all on their own— perhaps, speculate the researchers, by constricting arteries.*

Listen closely. Using a stethoscope placed inside your elbow and directly over the artery, your doctor listens carefully as the blood is released. The doctor listens first for a thumping sound—the sound of the heart as it contracts and pumps blood through the artery—and then looks at the pressure gauge for a reading. This is your systolic pressure, or the maximum pressure at which blood flows through your arteries. Then the doctor listens for the thumping sound to disappear—the sound of the heart at rest (between heartbeats)—and again glances at the gauge. This is your diastolic pressure, or the lowest pressure placed on your arteries.

Testing One, Two, Three...or More

No medical test is infallible, including the one for blood pressure. Many factors can influence a single blood pressure reading—what you ate that day, whether or not you're feeling rushed, any medications (including over-the-counter ones) you may have taken, and even your emotions at that moment the cuff is wrapped around your arm—like worrying about having your blood pressure tested!

Take talking, for instance. In one French study of people with high blood pressure, both systolic and diastolic measurements rose significantly while the participants gabbed away—and the pressure stayed elevated for a time even after the talking ceased. In fact, sitting quietly after talking was shown to be less effective in lowering blood pressure than reading a newspaper or a magazine.

➤**Pressure Point:** Because blood pressure readings can be inaccurate, doctors usually don't like to diagnose high blood pressure until you've been tested on at least three separate occasions. Having multiple measurements is especially important for people older than 65 because blood pressure tends to become more erratic as we age.

We're only human. Nurses and doctors can also make mistakes while taking a blood pressure reading. After all, no one's perfect. So if you think your blood pressure numbers don't add up—maybe they're drastically different than those taken at your last reading—then by all means ask for another test. Accuracy is very important because even a slight change up or down in either the systolic or diastolic pressure can mean the difference between a normal and high reading.

CAUTION

Intrigued by those small finger monitors for measuring your blood pressure—the ones where you simply stick your finger through a plastic ring and press a button? Don't waste your money. Readings from such digit monitors have been shown to be highly inaccurate. The same goes for those coin-operated blood pressure machines you sometimes see in malls and pharmacies.

Tips for Getting a Good Reading

- Allow yourself plenty of time to get to your doctor's appointment. Rushing can raise your blood pressure.

- Wear clothes that will easily let you expose a bare upper arm, so the cuff can be wrapped around it.

- Avoid caffeine, which can temporarily raise blood pressure, for at least 30 minutes before your reading.

- Don't smoke for at least 30 minutes before your reading.

- Rest quietly for about five minutes before your reading.

- Don't talk while having your blood pressure taken. Besides raising your blood pressure, talking makes it more difficult for the person doing the test to hear your heartbeat.

- Sit upright with your feet flat on the floor. Crossing your legs can affect your reading.

- During the reading, hold your arm out straight at about the same level as your heart. Better yet, rest your arm at heart level on a table.

- Make sure the right-size cuff is used. People with wide arms need wide cuffs.

- Make sure two readings are taken at each sitting. It's also a good idea to have a reading taken of each arm.

Number Crunching: What Your Reading Means

Both your systolic and diastolic pressures matter, which is why blood pressure readings are always described as two numbers. These numbers are usually written one before the other with a slash dividing them. The systolic pressure comes first; the diastolic pressure, second.

Blood pressure measurements are given in millimeters of mercury, which is abbreviated mm Hg. A 130/90 mm Hg blood pressure reading (spoken as "130 over 90"), means, therefore, that you have a systolic pressure of 130 mm Hg and a diastolic pressure of 90 mm Hg. Now, what do those numbers mean—in terms of your health, that is?

Optimal Numbers

If your systolic number is less than 120 and your diastolic is less than 80, then congratulations are in order! Your blood pressure is where health experts like to see it. Your numbers mean your heart doesn't have to strain to pump blood through your body and that your blood vessels appear in good working order.

But don't rest on your laurels. Like life, your BP changes. While it isn't a rite of passage that blood pressure creeps up with age, it does tend to in many cases. Continue following healthy habits and be sure to get your blood pressure rechecked within two years.

Normal Numbers

If your systolic number is between 110 and 129 and your diastolic is between 80 and 84, you're doing okay but not as well as you could. Your heart is laboring harder than it needs to, and it most likely has suffered some damage as has your blood vessels.

You need to take steps now—such as exercising more and eating more healthful foods—to reverse this trend and get your blood pressure back down to optimal levels. (These are the

BP to Go: The Take-Home Test

Measuring blood pressure at home sometimes becomes a key to evaluation and treatment. Rather than taking your own BP, a doctor will, in some cases, outfit you with a fully automatic portable device that is programmed to take your BP every 10 to 30 minutes over 6 to 24 hours. The results are stored in the device's memory. It is used when:

- Your doctor suspects that you had an artificially high reading in the office and wants to see if your blood pressure at home is normal.

- You complain of dizziness and other symptoms at certain times of the day and your doctor wants to see if your BP is responsible. Typically, this occurs during adjustments in medication or after introducing a new medication.

- You have hard-to-manage hypertension and your doctor wants to see how much your blood pressure fluctuates.

action steps you read about in Chapter 1; we'll be describing them in more detail later in the book.) You should also have your doctor recheck your blood pressure within two years.

High Normal Reading

If your systolic is between 130 and 139 and your diastolic is between 85 and 89, then you're standing on the precipice. You don't officially have high blood pressure, but your heart and arteries are definitely under added strain. You may even develop one of the serious problems associated with high blood pressure, including a heart attack, a stroke, or even a kidney disorder.

One study (of white Americans) showed that men with readings of 120 to 139/80 mm Hg were almost two and a half times more likely to die of heart disease than men with readings of less than 120/80 mm Hg. The news was even more dire for women: They were almost five times more likely to die of heart disease.

In fact, this category is a highly contentious one. Many experts believe its upper limits are too high. In 1999, the World

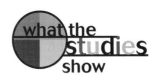

what the studies show

▶ *A study published in the* Archives of Internal Medicine *suggests that headaches may indicate Stage 1 or Stage 2 hypertension, which contradicts many experts' belief that high blood pressure doesn't have any symptoms. In fact, controlling blood pressure with medication reduced the incidence of headaches significantly.*

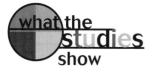

what the studies show

▶ *One study showed that 7 percent of men with Stage 1 high blood pressure had hearts with an enlarged left ventricle (the condition known as left ventricular hypertrophy). Another, much larger study of 5,500 men revealed that kidneys start to lose function when diastolic readings rise above 95 mm Hg. There's also good news: You can stop and even sometimes reverse the kidney damage by lowering your blood pressure—and keeping it there.*

▶ *According to the Framingham Heart Study, lowering your diastolic pressure by as little as 2 mm Hg can reduce your risk of stroke by 6 percent.*

Health Organization and the International Society of Hypertension recommended that the high normal limits be lowered to 130/85—which would mean that everyone in this category actually has high, not high normal, blood pressure.

You've got company. Perhaps the only thing "normal" about this category is the fact that so many Americans—an estimated 30 million—fall into it. If you are one of them, it's important that you focus on the high rather than the normal and make the lifestyle changes recommended throughout this book to sink your blood pressure levels. Also, be sure to have your blood pressure rechecked in one year. Here's a fact: Half of the people with high normal readings later go on to develop high blood pressure. Here's another fact: You don't have to be one of them.

Stage 1 High Blood Pressure

If your systolic is between 140 and 159 and your diastolic is between 90 and 99, then there's no longer any way of getting around it: You have high blood pressure. Doctors used to refer to this stage of high blood pressure as "mild" (and some still do), but don't be fooled. There's nothing mild about having any level of high blood pressure. Chances are, the pressure has already damaged some of your major organs.

So, take charge now. It's not too late to make a difference. Get your weight down, for example (if it's too high); shake the salt-shaker habit; cut down on alcohol consumption; exercise more; and so on. By committing to these things, you may be able to lower your blood pressure without medication and its potential side effects.

Also, be aware that Stage 1 high blood pressure can't be diagnosed from a single reading. Too many variables, from caffeine to stress, can influence your blood pressure during any given hour of any given day. Your doctor will want to check your pressure at least three times in order to get an accurate picture of your situation.

Stage 2 High Blood Pressure

If your systolic number is between 160 and 179 and your diastolic is between 100 and 109, you're in the danger zone. Your heart is undoubtedly becoming enlarged from

BP at a Glance: How Do You Stack Up?

Match up your latest blood pressure reading to the classifications in the chart below:

Classification	Systolic (mm Hg)		Diastolic (mm Hg)
Optimal	Less than 120	and	Less than 80
Normal	110 to 129	and	80 to 84
High normal	130 to 139	or	85 to 89
High Blood Pressure			
Stage 1	140 to 159	or	90 to 99
Stage 2	160 to 179	or	100 to 109
Stage 3	180 or higher	or	110 or higher

SOURCE: The Sixth Report of the Joint National Committee on the Prevention, Detection, Evaluation, and Treatment of High Blood Pressure, 1997.

Doctors used to base a diagnosis of high blood pressure only on the diastolic blood pressure. If it was over 90, you had high blood pressure, plain and simple. No one paid much attention to the systolic reading. In recent years, however, research has clearly shown that not only is a high systolic reading hazardous to your health but is also a more precise predictor of heart disease than the diastolic reading. Doctors now take both blood pressure readings seriously. You should, too.

pumping away at an exhaustive clip, and your arteries, too, are most likely showing signs of heavy wear and tear.

Doctors used to call this stage "moderate" high blood pressure, but few do anymore. And with good reason. Take the findings of just one worldwide study, which followed 13,000 men for a quarter of a century: Of the men with systolic readings over 160 mm Hg, 13.8 percent of those who died during the 25 years had suffered a stroke. Compare that with the men in the study with "normal" readings of 125 mm Hg: Only 3.2 percent of those who died had suffered a stroke.

Medication plus lifestyle changes. Your doctor will want to take more than one reading of your blood pressure before confirming that you have Stage 2 high blood pressure, so expect to make several visits to your doctor's office within the next month. He or she will probably prescribe medications for you immediately after the diagnosis is confirmed. But that doesn't get you off the hook for making several important lifestyle changes: Exercising, eating healthful foods, keeping your weight down, stopping smoking to name a few.

Stage 3 High Blood Pressure

If you have a systolic number that is 180 or higher and a diastolic of 110 or higher, you have a very, very serious condition. You are at great risk of developing heart disease,

Doctor Raise Your Blood Pressure?

If so, you're not alone. Some people's blood pressure goes up while in the doctor's office but is apparently normal at other times. This phenomenon has been dubbed "white-coat hypertension" (after the white lab coats doctors often wear) and is attributed to the stress and anxiety that people often feel during medical exams.

Although many experts consider the condition benign (when BP readings taken at home are normal), others think it's a warning sign. Researchers have found, for example, that :

■ people with white-coat hypertension have just as much plaque buildup in their arteries as people with persistent high blood pressure

■ people with white-coat hypertension are twice as likely to have left ventricular hypertrophy (swollen left ventricle of the heart) as people with normal blood pressure

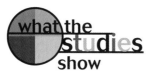
what the studies show

► *According to a study last year in the* Archives of Family Medicine, *Canadian researchers found that people with high blood pressure can actually have their BP reading go down in a medical setting—just the opposite of white-coat hypertension (see above). Such patients, the researchers conclude, are unlikely to be treated for HBP and therefore may miss out on the benefits of treatment.*

kidney disease, eye damage, and stroke. Your doctor will want to recheck your blood pressure and start you on medication immediately. Of course, you also need to make the lifestyle changes described throughout this book. Now. Today. Your life depends on it.

> **Pressure Point:** Medication can only reduce BP numbers so far. Many people have to embrace lifestyle changes as well.

Getting Behind the Numbers

The numbers are in, and they show you have high blood pressure. Now what? Unless you have extremely severe, or malignant HBP, your doctor will want to evaluate you more closely before sitting down and discussing a treatment game plan with you.

Why go to all this added fuss when the numbers make it clear you have high blood pressure? For three reasons. First, your doctor will want to determine if there's an underlying cause for your high blood pressure, such as a hormone imbalance caused by a growth on your adrenal glands, a kidney disorder, or perhaps a reaction to a medication. Remember, about 5 percent of people with high blood pressure develop the secondary type of the condition, which has a known—and often treatable—cause.

A damage estimate. Second, your doctor will want to thoroughly evaluate your health to determine whether your high blood pressure has damaged any of your organs, such as your heart or kidneys. And, finally, your doctor will want to figure out if you have any other risk factors that might increase your risk of heart disease and stroke—things like tobacco use, lack of exercise, high blood cholesterol, or diabetes.

Know Your History

Be prepared to field inquiries from your physician. He or she needs to ask you many questions to pinpoint what factors might be behind your high blood pressure and what risks you have for developing related conditions, especially heart disease. Be honest and open. You harm only yourself if you hold back any information out of embarrassment or fear of disapproval.

Contradictory Numbers: Now What?

Do your systolic and diastolic blood pressure measurements fall into two different categories? Then use the higher category to classify your condition. For example, if your blood pressure is 150/107 mm Hg, then consider yourself as having Stage 2 high blood pressure.

> Your doctor will probably start by asking you about your past health and about any present illnesses or conditions, as well as prior blood pressure readings.

> You'll also be asked about whether high blood pressure runs in your family and whether any close relatives have had stroke, heart problems, kidney disease, diabetes, high

cholesterol, or died prematurely from any cause. Don't leave out anything; all of this information is critical to your doctor's assessment of your condition.

> The doctor will delve into the details of your daily life, such as whether you smoke, how often you reach for the salt shaker, and how much daily exercise you get.

> He or she will probably also inquire about whether you're under any particular stress at work or at home.

> Other questions will center around the drugs you are currently taking. Be sure to tell the doctor about both prescription and nonprescription medications, including herbal and nutritional supplements. (Yes, that means vitamins, too.) Your doctor needs this information not only because many medications and supplements can increase blood pressure but also because some have a dangerous interaction when combined with some types of high blood pressure medications.

A Senior Moment

If your systolic blood pressure is higher than normal (140 mm Hg or above), but your diastolic pressure is in the optimal to high normal range (under 90), then you have a special type of high blood pressure known as isolated systolic hypertension (ISH). Most people with ISH are over the age of 60. In fact, it is the most common type of high blood pressure in this age group.

Doctors used to think ISH was a natural—and relatively harmless—consequence of aging, but now they know better. With ISH your risk of having a heart attack, heart failure, a stroke, or kidney failure rises dramatically. Fortunately, treating ISH can lower these risks.

Some people with ISH can get their systolic pressure down to normal levels through lifestyle changes alone. (Restricting salt and reducing weight have been shown to be particularly effective.) Talk with your physician about what's the best treatment plan for you.

Red Alert: Malignant HBP

If your blood pressure suddenly shoots up to very high levels, you are said to have malignant high blood pressure. This is a medical emergency and requires immediate treatment, perhaps hospitalization, to avoid permanent damage to your heart, blood vessels, brain, kidneys, and eyes. In fact, without treatment, the condition is fatal, usually within six months to a year.

A rarity but a real danger. Fortunately, malignant high blood pressure is rare. About 1 in 200 people develop it. The cause is often unknown, although the condition sometimes occurs in people who have a history of high blood pressure, particularly secondary high blood pressure resulting from a kidney disorder. You can also develop malignant high blood pressure if you abruptly stop taking your high blood pressure medication.

> Your doctor will also ask you about any symptoms that might indicate an underlying cause for your hypertension, such as headaches, excessive sweating, muscle cramps, excessive urination, or heart palpitations. For example, a swollen face and abdomen, headaches, increased thirst, and backache can be signs of Cushing's syndrome, an adrenal gland disorder that also spikes blood pressure.

Taking stock of your symptoms will help the doctor determine how much damage, if any, your high blood pressure has exacted on your body. Again, tell your doctor everything. A physical symptom that may seem minor to you—on-again/off-again headaches, for example, or a slight dizziness when standing up—may be an important clue to the status of your health.

Getting Physical: The Exam

According to one old saying, a good doctor has the observational abilities of Sherlock Holmes, the sensitive touch of an ace safe-cracker, and the ears of a rabbit. You can certainly expect your doctor to use all three of these skills—inspection (looking), palpation (feeling), and auscultation (listening)—during your physical

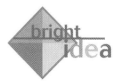

bright idea

▶ *Make a list of all the medications and supplements you are taking and bring it with you to your doctor's appointment. Or, if you prefer, bring the medications in their original containers.*

exam as he or she tries to determine a possible cause for your high blood pressure and signs of organ damage.

During your physical exam, your doctor may do some or all of the following:

Look in your eyes. Your physician will examine your eyes for retina damage. Twisted or leaky blood vessels in your eyes are also a good indication that other blood vessels in your body are damaged.

Listen to your heart. Using a stethoscope, your doctor will listen for sounds of possible heart disease—a fast heart rate, an abnormal rhythm, a heart murmur, or some other unusual sound. Because heart sounds can change when you change body position, your doctor may ask you to stand up, squat, or lie down as he or she listens to your heart.

Listen to your arteries. A stethoscope can also pick up what doctors call a bruit—the whispering sound caused by abnormally turbulent blood rushing through a narrowed artery. The most likely victims of turbulent blood flow are the carotid arteries in your neck, the abdominal aorta in your torso, the two femoral arteries in your groin, and the arteries on the inside of your thighs and behind your knees.

Listen for fluid in your lungs. Your doctor will listen through a stethoscope for the crackling sound of fluid in your lungs, an indication that your heart is working extra hard and inefficiently at pumping blood.

Feel your pulse. To assess your heart rate and rhythm, your doctor may take your pulse at a variety of locations in addition to your wrists. These sites may include:

➤ The inner part of both your elbows (the brachial pulse)

➤ Either side of your neck (the carotid pulse)

➤ Your abdomen (the abdominal pulse)

➤ The upper groin area of either of your legs (called the femoral pulse)

➤ Behind each of your knees (the popliteal pulse)

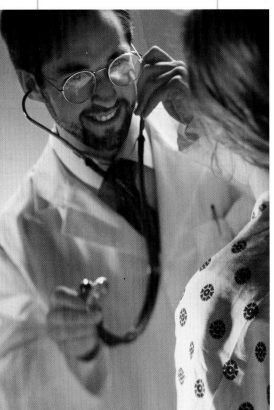

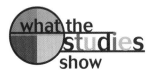
what the studies show

▶ *How do doctors decide what's ailing you? Research shows that 60 to 70 percent of the information doctors use to make a diagnosis comes from the patient's medical history.*

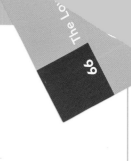

> On top of each of your feet (the dorsalis pedis pulse)

> On the inside of each of your legs, behind your inner ankles (the posterior tibialis pulse)

Your doctor will feel for a reduced pulse at each of these sites—an indication that the artery above the site may be possibly blocked or narrowed.

The Doctor's Office: Maximizing the Visit

■ **Be prepared.** Write your questions down ahead of time. Read them to your doctor before getting started. Also, bring a list of any symptoms you have experienced since your last visit. Include the dates that the symptoms began or stopped.

■ **Make eye contact.** You want your doctor to truly pay attention to what you're saying. Making eye contact with your doctor before you start talking can help get his or her thoughts out of your medical chart and focused on you.

■ **Speak up.** Don't be embarrassed to discuss sensitive topics with your doctor. He or she is trained to talk about personal matters with patients. And be sure to ask questions. If you don't understand something that is being said to you, tell your doctor and have it explained again to you.

■ **Tell all.** Holding back information—about symptoms you're experiencing, medications you're taking, or any other matter—is a dumb idea. The more information your doctor has, the better he or she will be able to diagnose and treat you.

■ **Take notes.** Write down the information and instructions your doctor gives you, or, if the doctor doesn't mind, tape-record what he says.

■ **Follow up.** If you forget something that was explained to you during the doctor's visit or if you think of a new question, don't hesitate to call the office. If you want to talk directly with the doctor, be persistent. The doctor may not be able to talk with you immediately, but he or she should call you back within a reasonable time.

Feel your abdomen. Your doctor will gently push on your abdomen for signs of an enlarged kidney or an aneurysm of the aorta, two possible consequences of high blood pressure. An enlarged kidney can also be a sign that your high blood pressure is the result of another condition.

Feel for swelling (edema). Swelling indicates an accumulation of fluid. Sometimes this fluid buildup is a sign of an underlying disorder; other times, it's an indication of a heart struggling to pump blood through hardened, narrowed arteries. Your doctor will look for swelling all over your body, but particularly in your face, lower legs, and ankles. To gauge the extent of the fluid retention, your doctor will press on your skin (such as over the ankle) and watch how far it can be pushed in and whether it stays indented.

Going into the Lab

The diagnosis of high blood pressure isn't arrived at lightly by your doctor. After all, you might have to take blood pressure medication for the rest of your life. This is serious stuff. So after taking your medical history and giving you a physical exam, your doctor may want to perform a few routine laboratory tests just to make doubly sure.

Urinalysis. Your urine will be checked for protein and blood—which are possible signs of kidney disease—and sugar (glucose), which can be an indicator of diabetes. Having diabetes makes controlling blood pressure more difficult.

> **Pressure Point:** High blood pressure often accompanies diabetes. This is because diabetes can damage your kidneys and cause them to retain water. More than 3 million Americans have both diabetes and high blood pressure.

Blood tests. A routine blood test consists of something called a complete blood cell count, or CBC, and an analysis of your blood chemistry. The CBC helps determine if you have an abnormal white or red blood cell count. Such abnormalities may suggest an underlying condition, such as anemia.

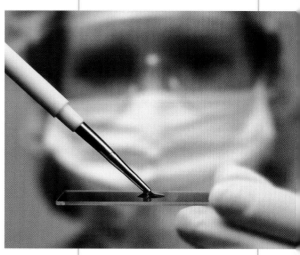

The blood chemistry analysis focuses on several key chemicals in your blood: sodium, potassium, calcium, protein, glucose, creatinine, and uric acid. High levels of potassium, for example, may indicate an adrenal gland problem; high levels of glucose may point to diabetes; and above-normal blood levels of creatinine or uric acid may indicate kidney damage.

The cholesterol-containing blood fats (lipids) in your blood will also be measured, including total cholesterol, triglycerides, "bad" LDL, and "good" HDL cholesterol. The higher your total cholesterol, "bad" LDL levels, and triglycerides, and the lower your "good" HDL levels, the greater your risk for heart disease.

Electrocardiogram (ECG). Used by doctors for more than 100 years, the electrocardiogram is a painless test that records your heart's electrical activity. Electrodes are attached to the skin on your chest, arms, and legs. The electrodes then transmit your heart's electrical impulses to an electrocardiograph, which records the impulses in the form of waves on graph paper.

This test helps your doctor check for signs of

> A heart attack

> An enlarged heart muscle

> Irregular heartbeats or rhythms

> An inadequate supply of blood and oxygen to your heart

And Even More Tests

Your doctor may discover something during your physical exam or as a result of your routine lab tests that causes him or her to recommend more specialized tests. The additional testing may be needed to confirm a suspected secondary cause of your high

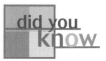

did you know

▶ *You may have heard an ECG referred to as an EKG. Don't be confused; they're the same test. The reason for the different acronyms can be linked back to Willem Einthoven, the Dutch physiologist who won the 1924 Nobel Prize in Medicine for his development of electrocardiograms. In Dutch, electrocardiogram is spelled "electrokardiogram" (abbreviated "EKG"). The English spelling has taken over in more recent years, although many doctors still say "EKG."*

How Low Can It Go?

Some people experience a sudden drop in blood pressure when they stand up that makes them feel light-headed or dizzy. They may lose their balance for a few moments or even faint. To check whether you have this potentially hazardous condition, known as orthostatic hypotension, your doctor will measure your blood pressure while you stand as well as while you sit.

blood pressure. Or, if you're already taking medication for your high blood pressure, your doctor may want to find out why your blood pressure hasn't dropped in response to it.

Here are some of the special tests your doctor may order:

A 24-hour urine test. As you would guess, this requires that you collect all of your urine for 24 hours. A laboratory will then check the samples for disproportionate levels of sodium and renin levels, a sign of renovascular hypertension, a common type of secondary hypertension that occurs when the arteries to the kidneys become partially or completely blocked. The laboratory will also check the urine samples for abnormal levels of certain hormones. Too much epinephrine in the urine, for example, can indicate a tumor in the adrenal glands.

Ultrasonography. This noninvasive technique uses high-frequency sound waves to obtain video pictures of your internal organs. It can show blood flowing through your arteries (to help find narrowing and blockages) and the size and shape of your kidneys (for signs of disease or deterioration). A special form of this procedure, known as echocardiography, enables doctors to observe details about the heart, such as its size, its pumping strength, and any damage to its muscle.

Computed tomography (CT scans). This X-ray technique can provide a detailed, three-dimensional view of your heart, kidneys, and other organs. The new ultra-fast CT scanners can look for increased calcium in your blood, an early sign that you may have blood vessel disease.

Magnetic resonance imaging (MRI). This technique (see photo below) uses magnetic fields and radio waves rather than X rays to produce images of your organs. A variation of the technique, known as magnetic resonance angiography (MRA), focuses on the arteries to get a good look at blood flow—and potential blockages.

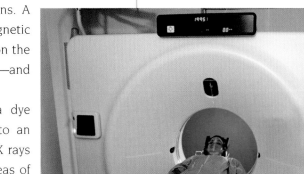

Angiography. In this procedure, a dye that's visible on X rays is injected into an artery through a fine tube, or catheter. X rays are then taken of specific arteries or areas of your heart. The procedure provides detailed information about the condition of these vital organs, such as how well your left ventricle is pumping and whether or where arteries are blocked by plaque or blood clots.

Nuclear scanning. This technique involves injecting a small amount of radioactive material in a vein, usually in the arm. A scanning camera then takes images as the material passes through a specific organ, revealing where damage has occurred. In the heart, for example, healthy areas take up and "show" the radioactive material while damaged areas don't.

Relieving the Pressure

Once your blood pressure readings are verified and your physical exam and lab tests are completed and analyzed, it's time for your doctor—and you—to team up to devise a treatment plan. A panel of experts from the National Heart, Lung, and Blood Institute doesn't recommend a dramatic rush to treatment but rather a gradual approach.

Lifestyle medicine. Unless you have Stage 2 high blood pressure or higher, treatment should start with lifestyle changes. That's right—medication is a last, not a first, resort for most cases of high blood pressure. Depending on what your health habits are right now, you may need to lose weight, become more active, eat more healthfully, reduce sodium and increase potassium in your diet, quit smoking, limit your alcohol, and control stress. This list should be sounding pretty familiar to you by now.

> **Pressure Point:** Everyone with HBP has his or her own unique disease. Some require only lifestyle changes; others require those changes plus medication. Some respond well to drugs that are ineffective in others.

Lifestyle changes may be enough to lower your blood pressure to safe levels. If not, however, you may need medication. At first you'll be given the lowest possible dose of a medication (probably a beta-blocker or a diuretic—more about the nine classes of antihypertensive drugs in Chapter 7), but if your blood pressure remains uncontrolled, your physician will gradually increase the dosage.

Piggybacking medicines. If after several months the first drugs haven't deflated your high blood pressure numbers, then your doctor will try other medications—perhaps an ACE (angiotensin-converting enzyme) inhibitor or a calcium channel blocker. Very stubborn cases of high blood pressure may require taking more than one medication at once.

Of course, all the time you're on these medications, you need

Time Off for Good Behavior

Taking medication for your high blood pressure? Wish you could go off it? Then stick with your healthful lifestyle changes. The people who are most successful at going off and staying off high blood pressure medication are the ones who are most aggressive at adopting more healthful habits. (Never, of course, go off any medication without first discussing it with your doctor.)

to stick with your lifestyle medicine as well. Why? Because medication alone is often not enough to lower blood pressure to optimal levels and because healthful habits build a strong heart and immune system, which will help your body fight off a host of diseases as you grow older.

You and Your Doctor: Still Talking?

In theory, it should be a fruitful, productive relationship, your doctor and you, but the facts would suggest otherwise. According to a recent survey of health care practitioners, doctors don't have the time to provide a meaningful explanation of high blood pressure. In the survey, patient-doctor communication received a woeful grade of D-plus.

Indeed, to adequately explain what hypertension is, its dangers, and how to live well with it takes more than the 15 minutes allotted for a typical doctor's appointment. So you need to pick up the slack by expanding your hypertension database—reading this book is an excellent start—and becoming a collaborator in, not just a recipient of, treatment alternatives.

Treatment plans should consider each individual as unique and different. No one method is considered best. The National Institutes of Health provides general treatment guidelines for high blood pressure management. But you and your doctor are given the responsibility of choosing a particular mode of therapy that is best suited for you.

One size doesn't fit all. Reducing salt may help a friend reduce her blood pressure but have little effect on yours. A particular medication may help lower your brother's blood pressure but do nothing for yours.

Obviously, you are the quarterback of your health-care team, your doctor is the coach, and your family members are the cheerleaders. It's essential that you be part of the treatment decision-making process. A big part. After all, you're the one—not your doctor—who will be donning those walking shoes at 7:00 A.M. each morning or remembering to take a pill once a day.

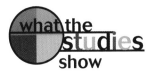
what the studies show

▶ *When patients with chronic health problems— hypertension, diabetes, and peptic ulcers—were coached on how to become more assertive with their doctors, they reported better overall health and fewer limitations on their social life and work life due to illness.*

The New Office Etiquette

Unlike arthritis, where the doctor's office might become your second home, high blood pressure lends itself to poor patient-doctor interaction simply because your visits are fewer and further between.

From passive to proactive. So you need to get involved. Before you decided to take charge of your high blood pressure, you might have just sat in the doctor's office passively, as your doctor asked you questions (or not) and told you whether you were doing well or poorly. How you felt was something you thought not worth mentioning.

Adopting a take-charge approach during doctor visits will help you get much more out of them. What would most benefit you—and would make your doctor happier—is for you to tell the doctor how you're doing: side effects from any medication you are taking, whether some of the lifestyle changes you are making are tougher than you thought, how you are feeling. And if you are having problems, you should volunteer the information and then spell out just what difficulties you are experiencing.

In fact, studies of people with chronic medical conditions (like high blood pressure) suggest that those who show the biggest health improvements are the ones who feel they have the biggest say in their treatment.

> **Pressure Point:** Only one-third of patients follow their doctor's treatment recommendations exactly as prescribed.

On the other hand, a uniquely silent disease such as high blood pressure is rife with patients who fail to take their condition seriously and are less than committed to making the lifestyle changes and, despite assuring doctors that they would, taking their medications. So thinking that you are doctor and patient is a mistake as well.

Second and third opinions. Although the majority of people with high blood pressure are cared for by primary-care providers, including family physicians, internists, physician assistants, and nurse practitioners, occasionally a medical consultation becomes necessary. The most common ones are:

> Dietitian/Nutritionist. These experts prescribe diets compatible with high blood pressure, diabetes, obesity, and other conditions. If you are hypertensive, your primary-care provider often will refer you to one of these nutritional counselors for low-sodium, low-cholesterol, or low-calorie diets.

> Ophthalmologist. Physicians who specialize in diseases of the eye, ophthalmologists will help treat damage to the delicate blood vessels of the eye or surrounding retina due to high blood pressure.

> Nephrologist. Internists with additional experience in treating diseases of the kidney, nephrologists usually treat people with secondary hypertension caused by conditions involving the kidneys, as well as those with untreated or undertreated primary hypertension whose kidneys have been damaged by the condition.

Whether you are working with just a primary-care physician or one of the above specialists, the approach is the same: Get in there and work closely with him. Let your thoughts be known. Do what the doctor orders, but make sure you have your input, too. Follow up and tell your doctor what's working and what isn't. In other words, insist on being an active partner in your health care.

You now know that high blood pressure is a serious condition. You also now know how you and your doctor can tell if you have the condition. Now it's time for you to find out in detail what you can do to lower your blood pressure and, equally important, to keep it there.

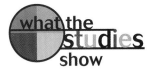

what the **studies** show

● *If you have diabetes, lowering your blood pressure will be especially good for your heart. Of the 1,501 patients in the Hypertension Optimal Treatment (HOT) Trial, those whose diastolic blood pressure was 80 mm Hg or lower had 51 percent fewer heart attacks and strokes than those whose diastolic pressure was around 90 mm Hg. The HOT findings suggest that people with diabetes should aim to get their diastolic pressure below 80 mm Hg and their systolic pressure at least below 135 mm Hg.*

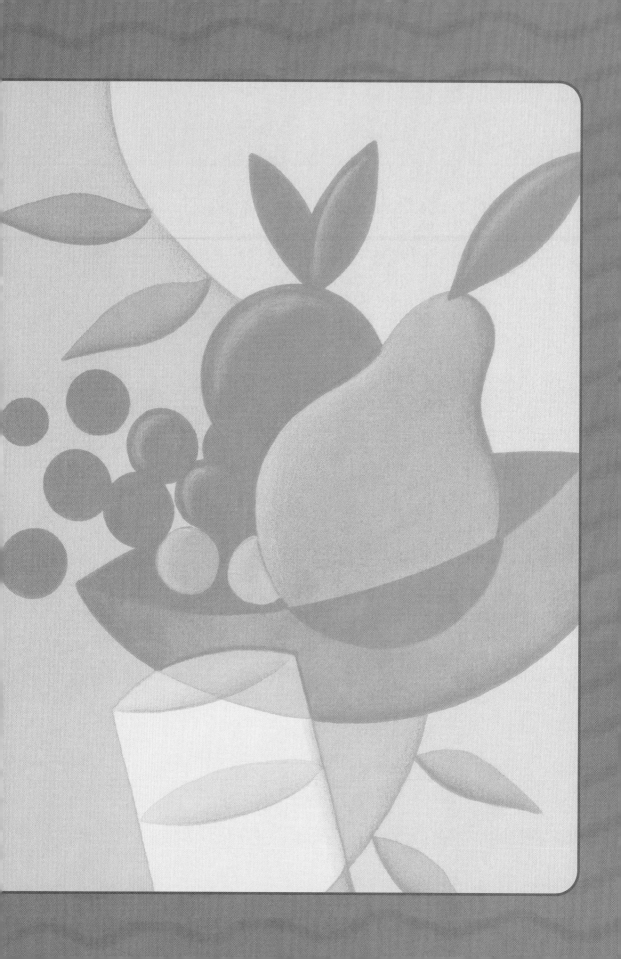

Fight Back With Food

Experts now know that the foods you eat

everyday can raise or lower your blood pres-

sure. Salt and fat can, over time, elevate your

pressure into the danger zone. A lot of fruits,

vegetables, and low-fat dairy foods can lower

it dramatically.

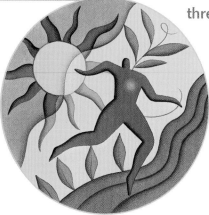

KEY CONCEPT You have to eat anyway, so take control of your three squares and help put a lid on your blood pressure. What's more, you'll feel and look better than you have in years.

The Importance of Losing It

If you're overweight and have high blood pressure, losing as little as 10 pounds may be the only thing you'll have to do to get your blood pressure back down into the optimal-to-normal range. No need to take medications. No need to cut back on salt.

You might not even need to reduce the stress in your life—although there are a host of other good reasons why you should. Sensible eating also holds benefits for those who don't have high blood pressure: For them, maintaining a healthy weight may be all they ever have to do to dodge the condition.

How can it be that simple? Because being overweight is a critical risk factor for developing high blood pressure. Studies have shown that carrying around excess poundage makes you two to six times more likely to have blood pressure of 140/90 mm Hg—or into dangerous high blood pressure range—than if your weight were in a healthy range.

A little means a lot. Nor do you have to gain a whole lot of weight to put yourself at risk for HBP. Just being pleasingly plump is enough. In 1998, researchers reported on a study involving more than 82,000 female nurses. They found that women whose weight crept up 11 to 22 pounds during adulthood increased their high blood pressure risk by 70 percent compared with women who stayed svelte enough to fit into the gown they wore to their high-school prom. The risk spiked even higher for women who gained more than 22 pounds.

> **Pressure Point:** You can drink wine and still get a beer belly. Studies have shown that it's how much you drink, not what you drink, that promotes abdominal fat—a risk factor for high blood pressure.

Given the fact that most of us in the United States pile on an average of 10 pounds during each decade of adulthood, this is bad news, indeed. Fortunately, when you take charge of your health, what goes up can also come down. In that same study of nurses, researchers found that women who lost 11 to 22 pounds lowered their risk for high blood pressure by 15 percent. And the women who worked hardest at counting calories and shed more than 22 pounds had even healthier results: a 25 percent drop in their risk for high blood pressure. Other studies involving men as well as women have had similar results.

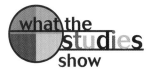

▶ *A summary of five different studies showed that losing 20 pounds decreases systolic blood pressure by an average of 6.3 mm Hg and diastolic blood pressure by an average of 3.2 mm Hg.*

Worth the Weight?

The truth is experts don't know exactly how excess pounds spike up your blood pressure. But they do. For instance, 40 percent of all people with hypertension are obese. The good news is that one in four hypertensives is able to control his or her BP by losing weight.

Although no one's absolutely sure why the extra poundage raises blood pressure, scientists have come up with several competing theories:

Theory 1: Most of the weight you gain is fatty tissue, which requires oxygen and nutrients just like the rest of your body. Extra capillaries have to be formed to shuttle the oxygen and nutrients to the tissue. In fact, for every pound of fat you put on, your body creates about one mile of new capillaries! Your body needs more blood for the freshly formed capillaries, and more blood means increased pressure on the walls of the arteries.

Theory 2: When you put on extra weight, your pancreas produces more insulin, which then lowers the amount of sodium you excrete in your urine. As a result, you retain more fluid in your body, which raises the volume of your blood—and your blood pressure.

The Problem with Pounds

Being overweight puts you at risk for more than high blood pressure—considerably more.

- Heart attack and stroke
- Some cancers
- Type 2 diabetes
- Gallbladder disease and gallstones
- Osteoarthritis
- Gout
- Kidney disease
- Cirrhosis of the liver
- Sleep apnea
- Low back pain

Theory 3: Carrying around extra fat cells simply puts too great a load on your circulatory system, causing your heart and blood vessels to work overly hard. The strain eventually becomes too much, damaging your heart and arteries and sending your blood pressure skyward.

The Weight-ing Game: Know Your Numbers

A few years ago, Americans got an unpleasant jolt when the National Heart, Lung, and Blood Institute issued new guidelines that lowered what's considered a healthy weight. Overnight, millions more Americans found themselves in the "overweight" category—and at risk for a host of medical problems, including high blood pressure.

The new federal guidelines (which are more in line with guidelines in other countries) use a formula known as the Body Mass Index (BMI) to determine whether or not a person is packing too many pounds. The BMI gives a much more accurate measure of body fat than simply standing on a bathroom scale—the standard, but now outdated, one-step method used for many years. The BMI does have some limitations, however. It tends, for example, to overestimate body fat in people who are very muscular and to underestimate body fat in people (especially the elderly) who have lost muscle mass.

Still, the BMI is a great tool for judging whether or not you're overweight. If you don't know your BMI, now's the time to find yours on the chart below.

The ABC's of the BMI

The Body Mass Index (BMI) is a calculation, not a direct measurement. It is figured by dividing a person's weight by the square of his or her height. Think of the BMI as a comparison of how much weight you're carrying per inch of height.

Height	Normal (BMI 19-24.9)	Overweight (BMI 25-29.9)	Obese (BMI 30-39.9)	Severely Obese (BMI 40 and over)
5'0"	97 to 127	128 to 152	153 to 203	204
5'1"	100 to 131	132 to 157	158 to 210	211
5'2"	104 to 135	136 to 163	164 to 217	218
5'3"	107 to 140	141 to 168	169 to 224	225
5'4"	110 to 144	145 to 173	174 to 231	232
5'5"	114 to 149	150 to 179	180 to 239	240
5'6"	118 to 154	155 to 185	186 to 246	247
5'7"	121 to 158	159 to 190	191 to 254	255
5'8"	125 to 163	164 to 196	197 to 261	262
5'9"	128 to 168	169 to 202	203 to 269	270
5'10"	132 to 173	174 to 208	209 to 277	278
5'11"	136 to 178	179 to 214	215 to 285	286
6'0"	140 to 183	184 to 220	221 to 293	294
6'1"	144 to 188	189 to 226	227 to 301	302
6'2"	148 to 193	194 to 232	233 to 310	311
6'3"	152 to 199	200 to 239	240 to 318	319
6'4"	156 to 204	205 to 245	246 to 327	328

Your fat-finding mission. Besides knowing your BMI, you also need to figure out where you're carrying most of your fat. Some people gain weight primarily in their hips and thighs, which gives them a "pear-shaped" figure. Others tend to carry extra pounds mostly around their waist, giving them an "apple-shaped" figure.

Research has shown that being a "pear" is better for your long-term health than being an "apple." Here's one big reason: People who accumulate fat around their waists—the "apples"—are more likely to develop high blood pressure. Scientists aren't exactly sure why "apples" tend to have higher BP, but it seems that abdominal fat is more likely to break down and gather in the arteries, where it can cause the kind of damage that leads to high blood pressure.

> **Pressure Point:** If you have an "apple" body type, you are at increased risk for Type 2 diabetes, heart disease, stroke, and certain types of cancer, as well as for high blood pressure.

What Kind of Fruit Are You?

To find out if you're an "apple" or a "pear," and whether you're carrying too much weight around your abdomen, measure the smallest part of your waist. Stand relaxed as you measure; don't "pull in" your stomach. You are at increased risk of high blood pressure and other health problems if:

- You are a man with a waist of more than 40 inches.
- You are a woman with a waist of more than 35 inches.

The increased risks are even greater if you also have a BMI of 25 or more.

Problem is, you can't change your body type—it's something you've inherited, like the color of your eyes or the shape of your nose. You are an "apple" or "pear" for life. So if you are an "apple," you should take extra steps to make sure you maintain your BMI at a healthy level (under 25). Watch what you eat and exercise regularly. (You'll find plenty of eating and exercising tips to accomplish both in this and the next chapter.)

And what if you're a "pear"? Well, don't think your body shape gives you free rein to gobble down french fries or doughnuts regularly. You still need to maintain a BMI of 25 or below to avoid high blood pressure and the other health problems that come with being overweight.

Counting Calories: What's Your Burn Rate?

The recipe for parting with pounds has been the same since the first Neanderthal noticed he had love handles: You need to eat fewer calories than you burn. You don't need to follow a fad diet; buy special, prepackaged meals; or invest in expensive exercise equipment. You just need to eat less and move more. Period.

Here's another simple fact about successful weight loss: In the end, it's the "tortoise," not the "hare," that wins. In other words, your goal should be to lose weight slowly and steadily— if you want to keep the pounds from coming back. Study after study has shown that the most successful dieters—the ones who reach and then stay at their desired weight year after year—shed their excess pounds gradually, over many months. They also permanently incorporate healthful eating and exercising habits into their daily routine.

Walk, don't run. Unfortunately, most dieters are "hares." Wanting to lose 10 to 15 pounds in a flash, they go on a crash diet, which sends their bodies into starvation mode, a complex biochemical response that results, initially at least, in lost water and muscle—not in lost fat. Worse, the body also downshifts your metabolism to a lower gear to conserve energy. So as soon as you go back to your old eating habits (and the vast majority of crash dieters do), your body begins to create even more fat than before.

Get a goal

So what's the best approach to losing weight? It begins with setting goals you can actually meet. According to diet experts (the ones not trying to sell you a book, a program, or frozen "diet" meals), your initial goal should be to lose 10 percent of your current body weight. And you should do it slowly, over a period of six months. For example, if you're overweight at 180 pounds (that is, if you have a BMI of 25 or more), you should aim to shed no more than 18 pounds over the next 24 to 26 weeks—very doable for most people.

Do the math. What does that mean in terms of calories? Well, if you have a BMI of 27 to 35, losing 10 percent of your body

Foods That Fill You Up with the Fewest Calories

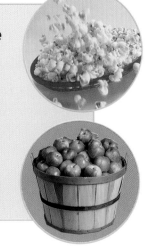

- Potatoes
- Fish
- Oatmeal
- Oranges
- Apples
- Whole-wheat pasta
- Grapes
- Air-popped popcorn
- Bran cereal
- Soup

weight will require taking in 300 to 500 fewer calories per day for a weight loss of about ½ to 1 pound per week. If your BMI is greater than 35, you will need to take in 500 to 1,000 fewer calories per day for a weight loss of 1 to 2 pounds per week.

> **Pressure Point:** Most weight loss comes from eating less rather than from exercising more. Exercise plays a big role, however, in preventing the pounds from creeping back on.

Let's translate those calories into "fast food," a language most of us speak fluently. The typical fast-food hamburger contains about 300 calories; a serving of french fries, almost 400; a milkshake, about 325; a single fried chicken breast, about 275; two slices of cheese pizza, 350 to 500; a bean burrito, about 450; and a 12-ounce container of soda, about 150. Even fast-food salad dressings are loaded with calories—typically around 300 calories in each packet (except for the light Italian dressings, which contain a mere 25 or so calories). So, as you can see, shedding 10 percent of your body weight over six months may require nothing more than giving up part of your fast-food habit!

Calorie calculus. Here is a quick and easy way for you to figure out how many calories you can consume each day and still lose about one pound a week. Multiply your current weight in pounds by 10. As an example: If you weigh 200 pounds, you should consume only 2,000 calories a day in order to lose a pound a week.

The long view

After six months, the rate at which you lose weight will probably slow down. It may even come to a screeching halt—the dreaded dieter's "plateau." Why? Because your body, at its new, reduced weight, expends less energy, which means it doesn't need as many calories. So to continue to lose weight, you need to further reduce the amount of calories you consume. And to keep from gaining back the weight you've already lost, you must be careful not to increase your calories.

If after six months you need to lose more pounds to get your BMI under 25, set a second realistic, long-term goal. Again, make sure it's no more than 10 percent of your body weight, and spread the weight loss over another six months. Remember, slow and sure wins the diet race!

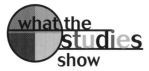

what the studies show

▶ *According to the Framingham Heart Study, people who are more than 20 percent over their ideal weight are eight times more likely to develop high blood pressure a decade later than people who are 10 percent under their ideal weight.*

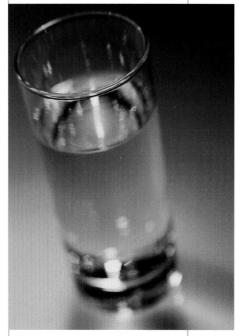

A Losing Formula: Ways to Lighten Up

The write way to lose. Start a food diary and record not just what you eat, but when and why you eat. Overeating is often triggered not by hunger, but by stress and emotions. You may eat to calm your nerves or to comfort yourself. Or you may reward yourself with food, such as when you've finished a difficult task. A recent survey of more than 1,000 adults revealed that nearly one-third of women snack out of boredom. Tracking the reasons behind your eating habits can help you develop more healthful behaviors. When you want to take a 15-minute break, for example, try taking a walk in a nearby park or get a quick errand done instead of munching your way through a bag of potato chips.

Partner up. Changing your eating habits and adopting a new, more vigorous exercise regime can be difficult to do on your own. Find a friend or family member who also wants to become a "loser." You can become a team and help motivate and inspire each other to keep working toward your mutual weight-loss goals.

Snack attack. Eating between meals can actually be a good thing. It can help maintain a feeling of fullness and reduce the temptation to binge during a meal. Of course, for your regular snacks you'll need to choose healthful, low-calorie foods—an apple or orange (instead of candy), a few pretzels (instead of cookies), or low-fat vanilla yogurt (instead of ice cream), air-popped popcorn instead of potato chips.

Nothing is verboten. Call it a dieter's law: The more you deny yourself a food, the more likely you are to eventually give in and binge on it. Any food can fit in your diet; just don't lose control and let the food torpedo your eating plan. Moderation and portion control should be the key.

Water power. Downing an eight-ounce glass of water a half hour or so before meals can help minimize your appetite. Sipping on water throughout the rest of the day may also help lessen your cravings for food. Several studies have shown that many people often eat or snack when they are actually thirsty, not hungry.

Freedom from fads. Gimmicky diets are not only hard to follow for a lifetime but also they often fail to provide all the nutrients your body needs to be healthy.

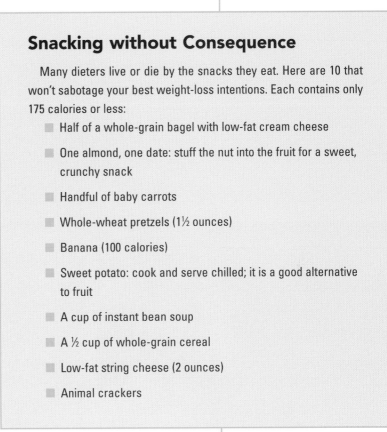

Snacking without Consequence

Many dieters live or die by the snacks they eat. Here are 10 that won't sabotage your best weight-loss intentions. Each contains only 175 calories or less:

- Half of a whole-grain bagel with low-fat cream cheese
- One almond, one date: stuff the nut into the fruit for a sweet, crunchy snack
- Handful of baby carrots
- Whole-wheat pretzels (1½ ounces)
- Banana (100 calories)
- Sweet potato: cook and serve chilled; it is a good alternative to fruit
- A cup of instant bean soup
- A ½ cup of whole-grain cereal
- Low-fat string cheese (2 ounces)
- Animal crackers

Some can be downright dangerous. Remember, no one food or product can quickly take off—and keep off—unwanted pounds.

The exercise prescription. Make time in your weekly schedule for 30 to 45 minutes of aerobic exercise (walking counts!) at least three times a week. Do muscle-strengthening exercises (such as lifting weights) another two days a week. And stretch every day. Studies show that the more adults exercise, the more well balanced their diet. (Chapter 4 will give you a rundown on incorporating exercise into your daily life and its relationship to high blood pressure.)

Be kind to yourself. Even the most motivated dieter "slips" from time to time and overeats. Also, be aware that some people, especially those with a family history of weight problems, simply have a more difficult time achieving their weight-loss goals. Don't berate yourself when your diet doesn't go precisely as planned. Just stay focused on your goal and get back on track.

DASH-ing to Lower Pressure

Even if you don't need to lose weight, adopting more healthful eating habits can help you lower your blood pressure—significantly. In fact, scientists reported in 1997 that the so-called DASH diet has the potential of being as effective as medication in lowering blood pressure. And the diet does it in about two weeks!

DASH stands for Dietary Approaches to Stop Hypertension, a study sponsored by the National Heart, Lung, and Blood Institute that was designed to figure out whether a diet rich in

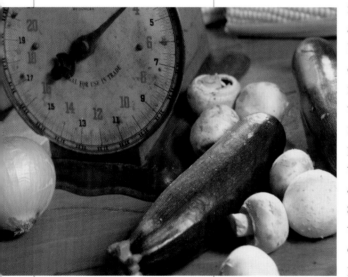

fruits, vegetables, low-fat dairy products and other reduced-fat foods could lower blood pressure. Here's how the study came about: The DASH scientists knew from earlier research that vegetarians tend to have lower blood pressure than meat-eaters. They also knew that most people—even those whose health is threatened by high blood pressure— aren't willing to veg out only on veggies. So the researchers decided to test a diet that mimicked a healthful vegetarian one—with a little meat thrown in to pacify the carnivores among us.

> **Pressure Point:** According to a survey by the Centers for Disease Control and Prevention, most 18- to 34-year-olds eat only one or two servings of produce daily. Forty percent of the over-65 set consume three or four servings. About 35 percent of seniors actually make it to five.

More than 450 men and women with average blood pressure readings of 132/85 mm Hg participated in the original DASH study. Many of them had high blood pressure (either a systolic pressure above 140 mm Hg or a diastolic pressure above 90 mm

Hg). One-third of the participants was put on a "typical" American diet, one low in fruits, veggies, and dairy products and with a fat content of around 40 percent of total calories. Another third was put on a diet that emphasized fruits and vegetables—at least eight servings per day—but it placed no restrictions on fat or dairy products. The final third went on a "combination" diet. It stressed fruits, vegetables, whole grains, and low-fat dairy products, but limited fat to less than 30 percent of total calories.

> **Pressure Point:** Scientists say that if more Americans adopted the DASH way of eating, there would be 15 percent fewer cases of heart disease and 27 percent fewer strokes.

The results, please. After eight weeks, the results were in: Both the fruit-and-vegetable diet and the combination diet lowered blood pressure. But the combination diet—what's now called the DASH diet—produced the most dramatic reductions. People on the DASH eating plan lowered their blood pressure by an average of about 6 mm Hg for systolic and 3 mm Hg for diastolic. Those people with high blood pressure fared even better. Their systolic pressure dropped, on average, about 11 mm Hg and their diastolic pressure about 6 mm Hg. And, perhaps most amazingly, the reductions came quickly—within two weeks of starting the DASH diet.

How does the DASH diet lower blood pressure? Scientists aren't sure. They think, however, that it may have a lot to do with the fact that the diet encourages weight loss. After all, the DASH diet recommends limiting the amount of saturated fat to no more than 6 percent—and your total fat to no more than 27 percent—of your daily calories.

As you probably already know, most of us eat too much fat, particularly saturated fat, the kind found in meat, full-fat dairy foods, and coconut and palm oils. The result: weight gain, clogged arteries, and a higher risk for heart disease and stroke. That's not good news for people with high blood pressure, who are already at increased risk for these health problems.

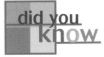

did you know

▶ *Scientists have proven that old adage, "Eat breakfast like a king, lunch like a prince, and dinner like a pauper." Studies have shown that calories eaten early in the day are less likely to turn into body fat than those consumed late in the day. Eat your biggest meal at breakfast, your next biggest at lunch, and your smallest at dinner. And, of course, eliminate those late-night snacks.*

The DASH diet also tends to be rich in potassium, magnesium, and calcium—minerals that have been linked in other studies to lower blood pressure. (More about these "miracle" minerals later in the chapter.)

On Your Mark, Get Set, DASH!

Getting started on the DASH diet is easy. You don't need any special foods or calorie calculators. Nor do you need to plan complicated meals or follow hard-to-understand recipes. (You will find a full seven-day DASH menu plan in the Resource Guide at the end of the book.) What you do need is to pay attention to what you eat. Specifically, try to work in the following types and amounts of foods into your life every day:

Grains: 7 or 8 servings

Grains include bread, cereals, rice, and pasta. Whenever possible, choose whole grains (such as whole-wheat bread and

The Skinny on Fats

Fats come in four basic forms—monounsaturated, polyunsaturated, saturated, and trans fats. Each has a different effect on your cholesterol (a waxy, fatlike substance found in your blood), your blood pressure, and on your risk for developing heart disease.

- Monounsaturated fat (found in avocados and olive, peanut, and canola oils) is the best of the three fats. It appears to reduce the level of the "bad" LDL cholesterol in your body and raise the "good" HDL cholesterol.

- Polyunsaturated fat (found in corn, cottonseed, safflower, soy, and sunflower oils) helps reduce LDL cholesterol, but it can also lower HDL cholesterol, which is not a good thing.

- Saturated fat (found in meat, dairy products, and coconut and palm oils) raises total blood cholesterol more than any other fat. Avoid it as much as possible!

- Trans fats, a highly processed vegetable oil found in margarines, commercial baked goods, and in oils used to prepare fried foods, may increase the risk for heart disease more than saturated fat.

Little Changes, Big Dividends

Want to lose weight? Think out of the box. Tweaking your diet, rather than banishing foods from the pantry, is the smartest approach around. For instance:

Meal	Instead of . . .	Try
Breakfast	Bakery bagel with 2 Tbsp of Cream cheese	2 pieces whole-wheat toast with 2 Tbsp peanut butter **Savings per day: 300 calories**
Lunch	Container of sweetened yogurt	Plain low-fat yogurt, ½ cup sliced fruit **Savings per day: 100 calories**
Dinner	Large plate of pasta (2½ cups) with ½ cup red sauce	4 oz. skinless chicken breast, 1 cup pasta and ½ cup red sauce **Savings per day: 240 calories**
Dessert	2 cups fat-free ice cream	Two miniature (0.7 oz.) candy bars **Savings per day: 200 calories**

brown rice) instead of refined varieties (such as white bread or white rice). Whole grains contain many more vitamins, minerals, fiber, and other nutrients. Refined grains—even "enriched" ones—are stripped of almost all their healthful nutrients. In fact, enriched white flour has only 25 percent of the potassium of whole-wheat flour.

Here are ways to incorporate whole grains into your diet:

> Start off your day with a whole-grain cereal (hot or cold), whole-grain toast or bagel, or whole-grain pancakes. For even more fiber and healthful nutrients, top the cereal and pancakes with fresh fruit and the breads with applesauce or other pure fruit spreads.

> Use whole-wheat breads for sandwiches and dinner rolls. But be sure to read food labels carefully when shopping for these items. Make sure the first ingredient listed on the label is "whole-wheat flour," not "wheat flour."

> add whole grains to the soups you make. Whole-wheat pasta and noodles make great additions to almost any vegetable soup, and brown rice adds taste and texture to bean soups and chili.

> Be adventuresome with your grains. Experiment with recipes that call for amaranth, buckwheat groats (kasha), quinoa, or whole-grain bulgur.

Fruits and vegetables: 8 to 10 servings

Not only are fruits and vegetables naturally low in fat and calories but they're also rich sources of vitamins (including potassium), minerals, fiber, and phytochemicals—substances that may protect you against heart disease and cancer. Here are some ways you can work more fruits and veggies into your daily menus:

> Buy a variety of fruits and vegetables when you shop. That way you'll have plenty of choices and you won't run out. First, use the ones that spoil the quickest, such as asparagus, bananas, and peaches. Save the hardier varieties, such as apples and winter squashes, for later in the week.

> At the office, fill a "fruit bowl" with raisins and other dried fruits and keep it within handy reach.

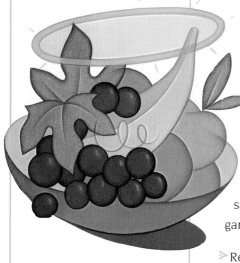

> For when you get the munchies at home, fill a bowl of cut-up fresh veggies and place on the top shelf of your refrigerator.

> Look for creative ways to add vegetables to your meals. You could grate carrots or zucchini into pasta sauces, for example, or toss steamed broccoli into a garden salad.

> Replace your daily dose of soda with fresh fruit juice.

Low-fat or fat-free dairy products: 2 or 3 servings

Milk, cheese, and yogurt offer plenty of protein and calcium. But these foods can also be high in fat. If you eat too many high-fat dairy products for too long, you're likely to develop an expanded waistline, clogged arteries, and elevated blood pressure. So be sure to choose fat-free or low-fat varieties, such as skim milk or low-fat yogurt. You'll get all the healthful nutrients without all the harmful fat. Here are some tips:

> Are you used to the rich taste of whole milk? Does skim milk seem thin and watery to you? Try giving your taste buds a chance to adjust to the absence of fat. Switch first to 2 percent, then to 1 percent, and then finally to skim milk. Soon you'll find that it's whole, not skim, milk that tastes weird. Or skip dairy and try soy milk.

> Choose cheeses that contain no more than two to six grams of fat per ounce. Most supermarkets now offer low-fat or skim-milk versions of ricotta, cottage, and mozzarella cheese. Low-fat farmer or pot cheeses also are available. The heart-healthiest cheeeses, however, are vegetarian ones made from soy protein.

> Use low-fat sour cream. Or substitute low-fat yogurt for sour cream in dips and toppings.

> Instead of ice cream, try ice milk, frozen yogurt (especially the fat-free variety), sherbet, or sorbet. If you do eat ice cream, opt for "soft serve" or "regular" rather than "super premium" types.

> Minimize the use of butter. Sauté in nonstick cookware.

what the studies show

> A recent study from Sweden suggests that vegetarians have lower blood pressure because of their fiber-rich diet. In the study, one group of participants received 20 fiber tablets a day while another group received a similar number of placebo tablets. Three months later, the diastolic blood pressure of the fiber-treated group was 4 mm Hg lower than in the placebo group. Interestingly, the fiber group also lost weight.

Don't Deny Yourself Dairy

If you have trouble digesting dairy products, now hear this: Most lactose-intolerant people can eat at least some dairy products as part of a meal but not alone. In addition, cultured dairy products, such as yogurt and buttermilk, are easier for lactose-intolerant people to digest. And there is very little lactose in cheese (it is removed in the process of cheese making), so it rarely causes a problem.

If you still have trouble with dairy products, add lactase liquid to the dairy foods at least 24 hours before eating to make them more digestible. (Lactase tablets aren't as efficient as the liquid.) You can purchase lactase enzyme products without a prescription at your local drugstore or supermarket. If you prefer, you can also buy lactose-free milk or milk that has lactase enzyme already added to it.

Meat, poultry, and fish: 2 or less

These foods are rich sources of protein and magnesium. But, like dairy products, they can be high in fat, and too much fatty food (as you undoubtedly know by now) can eventually lead to high blood pressure. So limit yourself to no more than two servings (3 ounces each) of meat, poultry, or fish each day. And try these ideas for cutting the fat:

> **Pressure Point:** Three ounces of meat is about the size of a deck of cards. When it comes to meat, think airline-size rather than restaurant-size portions.

> Select "lean" or "extra lean" cuts of meat. For lean beef and veal cuts, look for the word "loin" or "round" on the label. Lean pork cuts have the word "loin" or "leg" in their names. Trim all visible fat before cooking.

> Remove skin from chicken and turkey before eating. This simple action can cut in half the amount of fat in a serving.

> Refrigerate meat stews and soups. As they chill, much of the fat will rise and collect on the surface, where it can be easily removed before eating.

Not Hooked on Fish? Try Flaxseed

If you're a vegetarian who doesn't eat fish, you can still get heart-healthy omega-3 fatty acids by adding flaxseeds to your diet. Flaxseeds, like fish, contain high concentrations of omega-3s.

Because ground flaxseed goes rancid quickly, your best bet is to buy whole flaxseed and grind it yourself in a coffee grinder. Store the ground seed in the freezer, where it will last for up to six months. Use ground flaxseed in baking or in blender shakes, or sprinkle it on top of cereals and salads. One tablespoon per day is all you need. If you prefer, you can buy flaxseed oil. Use it in salad dressings, vegetable dips, and other dishes.

Eat more fish than meat or poultry. Most of the fat in fish is a "good" type known as omega-3 fatty acids. New research indicates that omega-3s may help lower blood pressure and protect against the formation of blood clots, thus reducing the risk for heart attacks and strokes.

Poaching, steaming, baking, or broiling are the most healthful ways to prepare fish. Avoid frying fish unless you use a nonstick pan or vegetable cooking spray. Also, don't serve fish with fatty sauces. Use lemon juice and herbs as a flavorful low-fat alternative instead.

Nuts, seeds, and legumes: 4 to 6 servings a week

Legumes (beans, dried peas, and lentils) as well as nuts and seeds are rich sources of plant protein and fiber as well as many nutrients, especially magnesium and potassium. Nuts and seeds also contain high concentrations of fat, although most of it is monounsaturated, the type believed to protect against heart disease. Still, try not to overindulge on nuts and seeds. Whenever possible, choose legumes instead.

> **Pressure Point:** You can substitute legumes for your daily meat servings. One cup of cooked beans gives you about the same protein as 2 ounces of meat.

Here are a few ways to include more legumes in your daily meal plan:

Open up a can of precooked garbanzo or kidney beans and add them to a salad.

Use nonfat canned refried beans instead of ground beef in tacos or burritos.

Cook up a big pot of bean or lentil soup; freeze it in small meal-size containers for lunches and dinners throughout the week.

bright idea

When you switch to the DASH diet, you'll find yourself suddenly eating more servings of fruits, vegetables, and grains than you are used to. All of that fiber may cause bloating and diarrhea. To help your body adjust, adopt the new eating plan gradually. Also, drink lots of water—at least eight 8-ounce glasses a day; fluids will help your body digest the fiber.

Added fats: limited amounts (2 or 3 a day)

Because meats, dairy products, and many prepared foods (even low-fat ones) already contain plenty of fat, the DASH diet recommends that you limit the fat (like mayonnaise, butter, and margarine) that you add to your meals to no more than three servings. Two servings would be even better.

Here's something to chew on: A single fat serving equals 1 teaspoon of margarine or 1 tablespoon of low-fat mayonnaise. Given that fact, how much added fat do you consume each day? Most likely, it's a lot more than two or three servings. Here are some tips to help cut back on added fat without sacrificing flavor:

> Use fats and oils sparingly—when cooking and at the table. Whenever possible, use nonstick pots and pans or vegetable cooking spray.

> Try sautéing foods in broth or bouillon.

> Flavor cooked vegetables, grains, meats, and other foods with herbs instead of oil or butter.

Clamping Down on Cholesterol

High cholesterol can be doubly dangerous for people with high blood pressure because it can further clog already-obstructed arteries, causing your heart to work very hard. The DASH diet will help because it is low in saturated fat—which causes your body to produce more cholesterol.

Two more things. But you can help matters further by decreasing the amount of cholesterol you eat every day. Fresh fruits and vegetables contain none; animal-based products like meats, eggs, and full-fat dairy products contain plenty.

Besides limiting cholesterol at its source, you can directly lower your current cholesterol levels by eating plenty of soluble fiber, found in oats, beans, peas, berries, apples, carrots, prunes, and pears.

> Use margarine instead of butter. Make sure the first ingredient listed on the label is water. Such margarines have one-seventh the amount of saturated fat of butter and one-third less trans fatty acids (molecules that lower "good" HDL cholesterol and raise "bad" LDL cholesterol).

> Use mustard on your sandwiches instead of mayonnaise.

> Enjoy dinner rolls without the butter. Use salsa or olive oil to increase taste appeal.

Sweets: limited amounts (5 a week)

Most of us gobble down far too much sugar—about 64 pounds a year, in fact. (To get a better picture of what that number means, imagine 13 five-pound bags of sugar lined up in a row.) Our consumption of sugar (which has been rising steadily for the past two decades) is one of the major reasons so many Americans are overweight. Sugary foods also squeeze healthier foods from our diets. If you drink nutrient-barren sugary soft drinks, for example, you're less likely to drink nutrient-rich fruit or vegetable juices.

The DASH diet limits sweets to five a week. Needless to say, you may find such deprivation difficult at first, particularly if you have a sweet tooth. But, believe it or not, sugar is actually an acquired taste. As you lower the amount of sugar in your diet, you'll find yourself craving it less.

Here are some tips for cutting back on sugar:

> Top French toast and pancakes with fresh fruit rather than maple syrup. To make the fruit "syrupy," cook it down with a little bit of water.

> Avoid flavored yogurts, which can contain up to seven teaspoons of added sugar. Instead, buy plain yogurt and add your own fresh fruit.

> Read cereal labels carefully. Avoid brands with added sugars. Sometimes the sugar is "hidden." Beware of ingredients that end in "ose," such as maltose and dextrose, as well as corn syrup solids. You guessed it: Those are sugars.

what the studies show

▶ Black licorice that contains glycyrrhinzinic acid, usually contained only in candy made from real licorice root, can raise blood pressure significantly. The chemical affects some of the hormones that regulate BP. Although red licorice doesn't contain the chemical, some dark beers, especially malt brews, add licorice as a sweetener.

DASH Diet: Day by Day

The serving sizes for the DASH diet are based on 2,000 calories a day. You may have to adjust the number of daily servings in a food group, depending on your particular caloric needs. You'll find a five-day meal plan in the *Resource Guide* at the back of the book.

Food Group	Serving	Serving Sizes
Grains & grain products	7-8 a day	1 slice whole-grain bread ½ whole-grain bagel, English muffin, or large pita bread 1 cup dry cereal ½ cup cooked rice, pasta, or cooked cereal
Fruits & vegetables	8-10 a day	1 medium apple or banana 12 grapes ½ cup raisins 1 cup raw leafy vegetables ½ cup cooked vegetables ½ cup (6 oz.) 100% fruit or vegetable juice
Low-fat dairy products	2-3 a day	1 cup (8 oz.) skim or low-fat milk 1 cup yogurt 1½ oz. fat-free or low-fat cheese 2 cups fat-free or low-fat cottage cheese
Meats, poultry & fish	2 or less a day	3 oz. cooked lean meat, skinned poultry, or fish 1 cup cooked legumes
Nuts, seeds & legumes	4-5 a week	1 cup (1½ oz.) nuts 2 Tbsp or ½ oz. seeds
Fats	Limited to 2-3 a day	1 tsp oil or soft margarine 1 tsp regular mayonnaise 1 Tbsp low-fat mayonnaise 1 Tbsp regular salad dressing 2 Tbsp light salad dressing
Sweets	Limited to 5 a week	1 Tbsp sugar, jelly, or jam ½ oz. (about 15) jelly beans 8 oz. lemonade 1 Tbsp maple syrup

The Shakedown on Salt

To salt or not to salt? That is the question for people with high blood pressure. And, until recently, there was no clear answer from the medical community.

Some people were directed by their doctors to lose the sodium; others could go ahead and eat salty dill pickles washed down with equally salty tomato juice. Now, thankfully, science has come up with a game plan for everyone.

Scientists themselves have been hotly divided on the issue for many years. Many believed that the best research showed a compelling connection between high salt—or, to be more accurate, high sodium—intake and high blood pressure; they recommended that some, if not all, people with high blood pressure restrict the amount of sodium in their diets. Other scientists, however, pointed to a countless number of studies published in the mid-1990s that indicated restricting sodium had only a minimal effect on blood pressure, at best.

(Remember, the more sodium in your blood, the more your blood volume increases—sodium attracts and holds on to water. As a result, your heart has to work harder to move the increased volume of blood through your blood vessels. The result? Increased pressure on your arteries.)

Then, early in 2001, came the results of a second DASH study. This study—dubbed DASH II—was conducted to look specifically at what would happen to blood pressure levels when people followed different diets with different levels of sodium. (In other words, the study was designed to try and end the "to salt or not to salt" debate once and for all.) The first DASH study hadn't tested salt reduction.

The 412 participants in DASH II were randomly assigned to eat either a "typical" American diet or the DASH diet. (To ensure against "cheating," all food was provided.) The people in both groups ate a high level of salt (3,300 milligrams a day—about the average American intake) for one month, a medium level (2,400 milligrams a day—the maximum recommended by the American Heart Association and other health organizations) for a second month, and a low level (1,500 milligrams a day) for a final, third month. About 40 percent of the study's participants

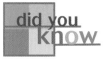

did you know

▶ *Most of us get only about 15 percent of our salt from the saltshaker at the dinner table. As much as 70 percent of the salt we eat every day comes from processed foods: cheese, soup, pretzels, spaghetti sauce, cereal, chips, bread, and many other foods.*

Deciphering Label Language

Do you know the difference between "unsalted" and "sodium-free"? If not, here is a rundown on what you'll find on food labels.

Sodium free	Less than 5 milligrams of sodium per serving
Very low-sodium	35 milligrams or less per serving
Low-sodium	140 milligrams or less per serving
Unsalted, no salt added, or without added salt	Made without added salt, but still contains the sodium that is a natural part of the food

had high blood pressure (blood pressure over 140/90 mm Hg); the rest had "high normal" blood pressure.

Low sodium, lower pressure. The study's results were astounding. They clearly showed that eating less sodium significantly lowers blood pressure—as much as taking a single blood pressure medication. The people in the study who consumed the least amount of salt—1,500 milligrams a day—experienced the most dramatic decrease in BP: an average drop of 8.9 mm Hg in systolic pressure and of 4.5 mm Hg in diastolic pressure.

> **Pressure Point:** A low-sodium diet may taste bland for only a few weeks. Studies show that as you use less salt, your preference for salt lessens. Most people adjust to lower-sodium foods in 14 days.

"Prior to our study, some experts had questioned whether it was worthwhile for people without high blood pressure to cut back on their salt intake," said Lawrence J. Appel, M.D., an associate professor of medicine at Johns Hopkins University and one of the principal authors of the study. "This study settles this controversy and further emphasizes the powerful effects of dietary change on blood pressure."

In fact, according to the National Heart, Lung, and Blood Institute, if Americans limited their salt intake to less than 1 teaspoon a day, strokes could be reduced by 42 percent and heart disease by more than 20 percent.

Do You Have a Salt Tooth?

So how much salt (sodium chloride) should you be eating? To begin with, you should know that your current diet is probably way too salty. You need no more than 200 to 500 milligrams of sodium a day—about the amount in ½ teaspoon of salt. Because sodium is found naturally in whole foods, from apples to broccoli to rice, you can easily get enough of it without ever picking up a saltshaker. And that's a good thing, because your body uses sodium to maintain fluid balance, transmit nerve impulses, and regulate your blood pressure.

But if you're like most Americans, you consume 8 to 10 times more salt than you need—a total of 4,000 to 6,000 milligrams a day. Measured in teaspoons, that's 2 to 3 a day.

Ah, you say, but you never salt your food, either when cooking or at the table. Well, that's a good start. But saltshakers account for only about 15 percent of the salt that lands in our food. The vast majority—nearly three-quarters—of the salt we ingest arrives "hidden" in processed foods. Canned vegetables and soups. Frozen dinners. Cheese. Pretzels. Potato chips. Cookies. Cakes. Breads. Breakfast cereals. Soft drinks. The list goes on and on.

Some processed and convenience foods are so highly salted, they deliver more than 1,000 milligrams of sodium in a single serving. One cup—just one—of many canned soups, for example, has well in excess of 1,000 milligrams. So does one deluxe fast-food burger, a couple of pieces of most pizzas, and several fried chicken breasts.

did you know

▶ *Before you try a salt substitute, check with your doctor. Some salt substitutes or "lite" salts contain a mixture of sodium chloride (salt) and other compounds. To achieve that salty taste, you may end up using more of the salt substitute than you do regular salt. The end result? You won't reduce your sodium intake at all.*

Less Salt and Less Fat: Doubly Effective

Lowering both the amount of fat and the amount of salt in your diet can be doubly helpful, as shown below.

Blood pressure status:	When on only a low-fat diet (no salt restrictions), blood pressure dropped:	When on only a low-salt diet (no fat restrictions), blood pressure dropped:	When on both a low-fat diet and a low-salt program, blood pressure dropped:
High blood pressure	3 mm Hg	8.3 mm Hg	11.5 mm Hg
High normal blood pressure	5 mm Hg	6.7 mm Hg	7.1 mm Hg

SOURCE: The DASH II Study, 2001

In general, the less processed the food, the less sodium is contained in it. One cup of whole-wheat flour, for example, contains 6 milligrams of sodium; a slice of whole-wheat bread contains 148 milligrams. A whole fresh peach contains 0 milligrams sodium; a piece of peach pie contains 253 milligrams.

Be a Sodium Sleuth

Sodium by any other name is still sodium. Here is a list of salty compounds you will find in many processed foods:

- Monosodium glutamate
- Baking powder
- Sodium bicarbonate
- Sodium propionate
- Disodium phosphate
- Sodium alginate
- Sodium benzoate
- Sodium hydroxide
- Sodium nitrate
- Sodium sulfite

Shed the saltshaker for good? Before DASH II, most experts recommended that people with high blood pressure consume no more than 2,400 milligrams of sodium a day (about 1 teaspoon). They also thought that only certain people with high blood pressure—perhaps half—were "salt sensitive," or likely to see their blood pressure drop if they cut back on salt. So they recommended that people cut back on their salt for a few weeks to see if doing so had any impact on their blood pressure. If the pressure dropped, the people were told to stay on a salt-restricted diet; if the pressure stayed the same, they were told not to bother.

Since DASH II, however, many experts are rethinking that game plan. The study showed that the more you cut back on salt, the greater the drop in blood pressure. So although restricting sodium to 2,400 milligrams a day is okay, limiting it to 1,500 milligrams appears to be even better. Furthermore, although the study confirmed that some groups of people—especially African Americans and women—benefitted the most from reducing the salt in their diets, every group, including young adults and even people without high blood pressure, saw their blood pressure go down when on a salt-restricted diet.

If you have high or even high normal blood pressure, you will probably benefit from eating less salt. How much you want to lower your salt intake is up to you and your doctor, but most experts agree that you should try to get it down to under 2,400 milligrams a day, at the very least. Fortunately, salt, like sugar, is an acquired taste. The less you eat of it, the less you'll crave it.

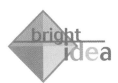

CAUTION

For most people, reducing salt is a good thing. But for a few, it can be dangerous. Some people with certain kidney diseases, for example, have trouble maintaining healthy sodium levels in their body. If you have kidney problems, talk with your doctor before making a major change in your diet.

Shaking Salt from Your Diet

> Eat fewer processed or "convenience" foods. Whole foods, like fresh fruits and vegetables, are naturally low in salt.

> When you do buy processed foods, read labels carefully. Look for unsalted or low-sodium varieties.

> Don't cook with salt. If you must add salt, do so at the end; you'll need much less of it. Salty flavor becomes muted the longer a food cooks.

> Flavor your meals with herbs, spices, lemon, lime, or vinegar instead of salt.

> When eating out, request that the chef omit salt from your meal. Many restaurants will honor such a request.

> Plan ahead. If you know your dinner will be high in salt, make your breakfast and lunch "no-sodium" meals.

bright idea

▶ *Keep a sodium diary. Read food labels for sodium content and note how much salt you add to your foods, both in the kitchen and at the table. Write down the amounts in a small notebook. You may be surprised at how much sodium you consume each day. Your diary should also help you decide how you can best shake salt from your diet.*

Mind Your Minerals

Several minerals may be just as important as salt in regulating blood pressure. Scientists are pretty sure that one of them—potassium—can be used to help lower blood pressure. Exactly what role the other two—calcium and magnesium—play in the treatment of high blood pressure remains to be determined.

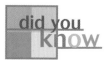

did you know

▶ *African Americans, whose diets tend to be very low in potassium, may especially benefit from increasing potassium levels. One study showed a remarkable drop of 20 mm Hg in systolic pressure and a drop of 13 mm Hg in diastolic pressure for African Americans taking potassium pills.*

Pass the Potassium, Please

It's very simple: If your body is low in potassium, your blood pressure is likely to go up. Recent studies have also shown that eating a potassium-rich diet—or taking potassium supplements—can reduce blood pressure. The potassium appears to lower blood pressure by creating a healthy balance of sodium in your cells. In fact, potassium is the third most abundant mineral in the body after calcium and phosphorus; almost all of the potassium in the body is found inside the cells.

A coming-out party. The spotlight shone on potassium as a potential aid in treating high blood pressure in 1997, when a group of scientists analyzed the findings of 33 different randomized studies. This meta-analysis found that people with high blood pressure who took potassium supplements had an average drop in systolic pressure of 4.4 mm Hg and in diastolic pressure of 2.5 mm Hg. People with normal blood pressure had an average drop of 2 mm Hg in systolic pressure and 1 point in diastolic. These small changes reduce the chance of developing hypertension by 25 percent.

In general, aim to consume about 3,500 milligrams of potassium a day. Your best bet is simply to eat more potassium-rich foods, especially fruits, vegetables, and low-fat dairy products. If you're following the DASH diet, eating these foods shouldn't be much of a problem. Have a cup of orange juice with breakfast, half an avocado in a salad at lunch, and half a cup of cooked spinach or a baked potato with dinner. For snacks, try a banana, 8 ounces of low-fat yogurt, or five dried prunes.

> **Pressure Point:** Microwave or steam vegetables whenever possible—boiling them decreases their potassium content. A boiled potato, for example, loses 50 percent of its potassium; steamed potatoes lose less than 6 percent.

You might also want to consider taking potassium supplements, particularly if you're having trouble limiting the salt in your diet; the supplements seem to help mediate the bad effects of too much salt in the body. (But don't think that by adding potassium to your diet you can reinstate the salt-shaker to your dinner table!) If you're taking a class of blood pressure drugs called diuretics, your doctor may recommend potassium supplements. Diuretics flush extra salt and water from the body, and sometimes potassium goes along for the ride. (Find out more about diuretics in Chapter 7.)

Below you will find foods that contain plentiful amounts of potassium (starting with those that contain the greatest amounts of the mineral). Don't just home in on the best-sources of the mineral; eating a wide range of foods provides healthy benefits, like phytochemicals and fiber.

> ### CAUTION
>
> Not everyone should stockpile potassium. There are some who should beware. For instance:
>
> ✦ People with high blood pressure who take certain medications, such as potassium-sparing diuretics or ACE inhibitors, are also at risk of developing heart problems if they take in too much of the mineral.
>
> ✦ People suffering from kidney problems or with kidney disease.
>
> In either case, be sure to talk with your doctor before upping the amount of potassium in your diet.

- **Apricots, dried:** 1 cup, 1,567 mg

- **Avocado:** 1 medium, 1,097 mg

- **Potato (baked with skin):** 1 medium, 844 mg

- **Pinto beans:** 3 oz. cooked, 646 mg

- **Yogurt:** 8 oz., 579 mg

- **Orange juice:** 1 cup, 550 mg

- **Cantaloupe:** 1 cup, 482 mg

- **Banana:** 1 medium, 467 mg

- **Winter squash:** ½ cup cooked, 448 mg

- **Spinach:** ½ cup cooked, 419 mg

- **Lima beans:** ½ cup cooked, 354 mg

- **Prunes (dried):** ½ cup, 317 mg

- **Raisins:** ½ cup, 310 mg

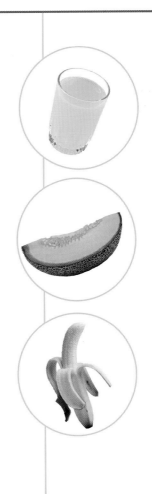

Can You Count on Calcium?

Here's what we know for sure (sort of) about calcium: Having too little of the mineral in our bodies seems to increase our risk for high blood pressure. Take the findings from the study of 80,000-plus American nurses, known as the Nurses' Health Study. Women in that study who consumed at least 800 milligrams of calcium daily had a 23 percent lower risk for high blood pressure than women who ingested less than 400 milligrams of calcium.

Pregnancy: The Calcium Effect

Getting enough calcium during pregnancy can cut in half a mother-to-be's risk of developing pregnancy-induced high blood pressure. Studies have also shown that women with good stores of calcium tend to have babies with higher birth rates and lower blood pressure. How much calcium do you need during pregnancy? Doctors recommend 1,500 to 2,000 milligrams daily.

You would think, therefore, that popping calcium supplements every day would help reduce blood pressure. But, unfortunately, studies have shown that not to be true. Calcium supplements have little, if any, impact on blood pressure.

> **Pressure Point:** Although calcium is the most abundant mineral in the body, most adults get just half the calcium they need each day.

Still, given that a deficiency of calcium has been linked to high blood pressure, don't take chances. Make sure you get enough of the mineral. If you're under age 50, you should be taking in at least 1,000 milligrams of calcium a day; if you're over age 50, bump that amount up to 1,200 milligrams (for men) or 1,500 (for women).

Foods first. Try to get most of your calcium from food sources rather than supplements. Dairy products are particularly high in calcium—an 8-ounce glass of milk, for example, contains about 300 milligrams of the mineral—but they can also be loaded with fat. So be sure to follow the DASH dictum: Always choose fat-free or low-fat milk, cheese, and yogurt. And go very easy on the butter.

Below you will find the foods that are most plentiful in the mineral calcium. Once again, try to eat all of the foods rather than focusing on just the richest sources.

- **Yogurt (plain, fat-free):** 1 cup, 400 mg

- **Collard greens (cooked):** 1 cup, 357 mg

- **Ricotta cheese (part skim):** ½ cup, 337 mg

- **Milk (fat-free or low-fat):** 1 cup, 300 mg

- **Orange juice (with added calcium):** 1 cup, 300 mg

- **Tofu (processed with calcium sulfate):** ½ cup, 260 mg

- **Broccoli (cooked):** 1 cup, 118 mg

- **Almonds (dry roasted):** ½ cup, 100 mg

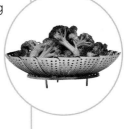

C—It Works

You've probably heard of vitamin C as a possible preventive treatment for the common cold, but will it also protect against high blood pressure? Yes, according to a recent study. In Boston, researchers gave one group of people with high blood pressure daily doses of 500 milligrams of vitamin C and another group placebo pills. One month later, the average blood pressure of the people who took the vitamin C had dropped 9.1 percent compared to 2.7 percent for the people in the placebo group.

How it works. The study's authors believe vitamin C may lower blood pressure by maintaining the body's supply of nitric oxide, needed for blood vessels to relax. When blood vessels tighten, blood pressure goes up; when they relax, blood pressure goes down.

Getting vitamin C from foods is easy—one cup of orange juice contains 124 milligrams of the nutrient. Other good food sources include green peppers, broccoli, tomatoes, and strawberries.

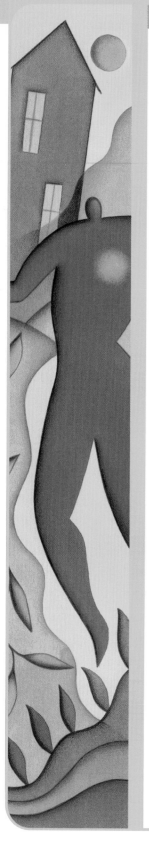

REAL-LIFE MEDICINE

Meals That Heal: One Man's Food Fight

Cleveland Sample, 72, was a General Motors production superintendent. He was responsible for 1,300 workers and had other things on his mind than cooking. Then, during an annual physical, the doctor said his blood pressure was 150/90 mm Hg.

"I didn't think it could happen to me," says Sample, who hails from Ellicott City, Maryland. "I didn't smoke or drink, and high blood pressure wasn't in my family—no more than most African-American families."

The doctor advised losing weight, exercising, and reducing job stress. "Didn't work," he says, and two years after diagnosis he began taking medication.

One day after work, a newspaper ad caught Sample's eye. A nearby hospital sought subjects for a study on diet and hypertension. He immediately enrolled, he says, because "rather than taking medication, I wanted to control my blood pressure naturally."

Sample met with other study subjects once a week for 18 months. He learned to prepare foods using seasonings other than salt. "I didn't go cold-turkey on eating less salt. I did it more gradually. I just have to have salt with my eggs. So I would still have it, but instead of having two eggs I'd have one." Sample stopped taking medication, and still his blood pressure fell to 130/75. Eating more fish and poultry helped his weight drop from 193 to 180 pounds. "And I started to cook," he says. "I was the one with the problem, and if I wanted something specific to eat, I'd fix it myself."

Over the years, Sample's blood pressure has stayed down, thanks to low-dosage medication and his careful but creative cooking. Try sampling his stir-fry: Place pork, beef, shrimp, chicken, or scallops in a marinade of garlic, ginger, cornstarch, and peanut oil. Then stir-fry the meat or fish with plenty of vegetables and a little low-sodium soy sauce.

"I like that I'm not at the mercy of someone or something else when I cook," says Sample. "I can fix what I need to maintain my own health."

> **"I wanted to control my BP naturally," says Cleveland Sample.**

Magnesium Is a Maybe

As with calcium, having too little magnesium has been linked to high blood pressure. Some studies have also shown that taking magnesium supplements can lower blood pressure slightly, particularly in people whose blood pressure is over 140/90 mm Hg. But findings haven't been consistent, and most experts remain unconvinced of the value of prescribing magnesium willy-nilly to people with high blood pressure.

Mining magnesium. Still, you might as well make sure you're getting enough of this important mineral. After all, one of magnesium's many duties in the body is increasing the width of blood vessels, a task that may explain how it helps knock down blood pressure.

The recommended daily dose of magnesium is 400 milligrams. Once again, remember that nature is best—and cheaper. Try to get the nutrient naturally through foods rather than through supplements.

Below you will find foods that are rich in magnesium. Try all of the foods rather than focusing on just the richest sources of the mineral.

- **Almonds or hazelnuts:** 2 oz., 170 mg

- **Spinach (cooked):** 1 cup, 155 mg

- **Swiss chard (cooked):** 1 cup, 150 mg

- **Sunflower seeds (dried):** ½ cup, 130 mg

- **Halibut or mackerel (cooked):** 4 oz., 120 mg

- **Tofu:** 4 oz.,120 mg

- **Brown rice (cooked):** 1 cup, 85 mg

- **Avocado:** 6 oz., 70 mg

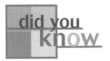
did you know

▶ *Research shows that magnesium citrate is the form most readily absorbed by the body. Magnesium oxide may be the least expensive, but it's also the most poorly absorbed.*

4 The Exercise Prescription

There is little that exercise doesn't help,

including high blood pressure. Getting

physical is one of the most effective ways

to chase away pounds, strengthen your ticker,

create more elastic blood vessels, and reduce

stress and tension—a four-part recipe for

helping to lower BP levels.

Exercise is the essence of the take-charge approach: It is inexpensive, readily available, free from the side effects associated with medications—and a choice only you can make.

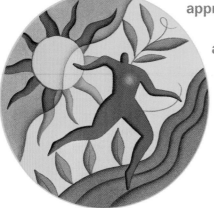

Are You Getting Enough Vitamin X?

When it comes to lowering blood pressure and bolstering your heart, regular exercise—known, in some circles, as vitamin X—is a prescription for success. Studies have repeatedly shown that daily physical activity can lower blood pressure—sometimes as effectively as high blood pressure medications.

And what if you don't have high blood pressure and your goal is simply to keep things that way? Regular exercise is also great preventive medicine: It can help put a lid on your blood pressure, so that it never reaches heart-damaging levels.

The road not taken. For many of us, exercise is the prescription that never gets written. Only about 22 percent of Americans get at least 30 minutes of moderate physical activity most days—the minimum requirement, say the experts, for effectively lowering high blood pressure and protecting the heart. Among that 22 percent are the determined walkers you see circling your neighborhood early each morning; the daily swimmers who glide through lap after lap at your local YMCA; the home-gym enthusiasts who work out while watching the evening news. And many, many others.

But what about the rest of us? About 54 percent of American adults get some exercise, but they don't do it regularly or intensely enough to reap any cardiovascular benefits. They may walk or swim or ride a stationary bike, but only sporadically. Then there are the 25 percent of Americans over the age of 18 (38 percent over the age of 55) who are totally inactive. They get no meaningful physical activity whatsoever. Zilch.

Combine the people who never get moving with those who barely do so and you have a depressing statistic: About 80 percent of Americans are so inactive that it threatens their health.

Movement Matters

Try as you may, you can't deny the volumes of research extolling the benefits of exercise. Study after study has shown that physical inactivity is a major risk factor for high blood pressure and heart disease. Less-fit people have a 30 to 50 percent greater risk for developing high blood pressure than those who hit the treadmill or strength-train regularly. They are also two-and-a-half times more likely to develop heart disease. Physical inactivity also raises the risk for developing diabetes, several cancers, and a host of other serious health problems.

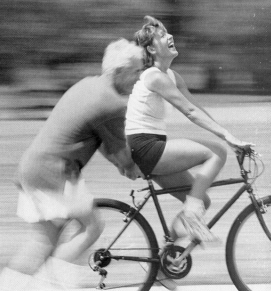

All in all, up to 250,000 deaths per year—or 12 percent of all deaths—in the United States are due to lack of regular physical activity.

How exercise sinks BP. To begin with, regular exercise helps you shed excess pounds, which, as we talked about in Chapter 2, can significantly lower blood pressure. It's common sense: Any time you burn more calories than you consume, you lose weight. Exercise fuels the body's furnace, so that more of the calories are burned, not stored. In fact, unless you include exercise in your weight-loss plan, you'll have a hard time achieving—and perhaps an impossible time maintaining—a healthy weight.

But losing enough excess baggage to go from a size 10 to a size 8 isn't the only reason exercisers experience a drop in blood pressure. Several studies have shown that regular physical activity sometimes sends blood pressure downward even if you don't lose a single pound. Doctors aren't sure why, but they think this phenomenon may well be linked to the positive effect exercise seems to have on the heart and circulatory system.

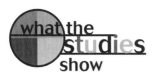

◑ *A single 45-minute session on a treadmill is enough to significantly reduce both systolic and diastolic blood pressure for many hours, according to a study by researchers at the University of Maryland. The researchers had 11 obese men, ranging in age from 49 to 67, walk for three 15-minute sessions on a treadmill, with four-minute "breaks" in between. Systolic blood pressure dropped from 6 to 13 mm Hg and diastolic pressure from 4 to 8 mm Hg right after the exercise session. Here's the kicker: The blood pressure stayed down for about 24 hours.*

➤ **Pressure Point:** Scientists now think that 80 percent of the health problems once associated with growing old— including high blood pressure—can be prevented, or at least postponed, by staying fit.

The more physically fit you are, the stronger and more efficient your heart muscle and lungs become. In addition, a sweaty session of exercise also works wonders in the arteries: New studies have shown that regular exercise helps maintain healthy, "young" blood vessels. In fact, physically active 60-year-olds have been found to have arteries similar to 40-year-olds.

What's the secret? Exercise apparently prevents the lining of the blood vessels, known as the endothelium, from deteriorating and hardening, thus staving off the development of plaque blockages and blood clots. Also, the healthier the endothelium, the easier it is for blood vessels to relax and allow blood to flow through. Exercise also helps to increase HDL ("good") cholesterol, which ushers LDL ("bad") cholesterol out of your body. Add it all up, and exercise does an exceptional job of reducing strain on your entire circulatory system.

Convinced yet that exercise should be part of your high blood pressure prescription? We thought so. Well, let's get moving.

Aerobics: Putting the Moves on Your HBP

Some people call them isotonic exercises, others refer to them as dynamic exercises, but most of us call them good ol' aerobics. Whatever you call them, they are the best kind of activities for knocking down your blood pressure numbers.

Exercises that elevate your heart rate are considered aerobic. To be technical about it for a moment, aerobic exercise is any activity that uses the body's large muscles—usually your leg

The Original Anti-Aging Pill

Want to live longer and feel better as you do so? Then do some kind of activity every day. According to the Centers for Disease Control, regular physical activity:

▓ Reduces the risk of dying prematurely

▓ Reduces the risk of dying from heart disease

▓ Reduces the risk of developing diabetes

▓ Reduces the risk of developing high blood pressure

▓ Helps reduce blood pressure in people who already have high blood pressure

▓ Reduces the risk of developing colon cancer

▓ Reduces feelings of depression and anxiety

▓ Helps control weight

▓ Helps build and maintain healthy bones, muscles, and joints

▓ Helps older adults become stronger and better able to move about without falling

▓ Promotes psychological well-being

muscles—in a repetitive fashion long enough to get your heart beating at 60 to 80 percent of its maximum rate for at least 20, but preferably, 30 minutes.

Most importantly, aerobic exercises condition your heart to pump efficiently so that oxygen can be transmitted to your working muscle cells. (Aerobic means "with oxygen.") Virtually any activity—brisk walking, running, bicycling, skating, swimming—qualifies as aerobics if it meets the above definition.

Exercise without the sweat. What you may not know, however, is that aerobic activities can also sometimes include nonsporting activities, like gardening and ballroom dancing. In fact, studies have shown that lower-gear moderate exercise extends many of the same health benefits to your heart and circulatory system that full-throttle activities do.

For an activity to "count" as an aerobic one, however, it must be done with an intensity for a long enough time to give your heart and lungs a reasonable workout. The activity must also be done frequently if it is going to have any long-lasting effect on your cardiovascular system. You must consider all three of these features—intensity, duration, and frequency—when planning your personal exercise strategy.

> **▷Pressure Point:** In terms of overall health benefits, it doesn't matter what you do to get in shape as long as you burn at least 1,000 to 2,000 calories a week in activity.

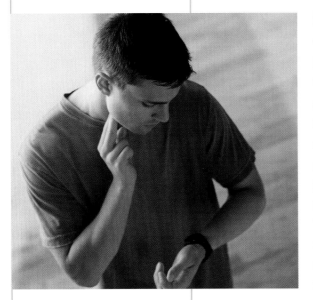

How Intense?

The more intense an activity, the faster your heart beats—and the more benefit you get. When you're beginning an exercise program, you should aim for working out at an intensity that is 50 to 70 percent of your maximum heart rate. Experts refer to this pace as "moderately intense." Gradually, as you get in better shape, you can increase the intensity of your workouts to between 70 and 85 percent of your maximum heart rate. (These ranges are just suggestions. Be sure to talk with your doctor about what intensity is right for you.)

Know your max

How can you tell if you've reached the desired intensity during a workout? First, you have to know your maximum heart rate. Just do this simple calculation: Subtract your age from the number 220. If you are 50 years old, for example, your maximum heart rate—or pulse—would be 170 beats per minute (220 minus 50 equals 170).

Next, multiply your maximum heart rate by .50 and .70 (for a moderate workout) or .70 to .85 (for a vigorous one). Those numbers are the lower and upper ranges of what your pulse should be during each kind of workout. In other words, if you're 50 years old, your pulse should beat at a rate of 85 (.50 x 170) to 119 (.70 x 170) times per minute during a moderately intense workout; if you want a vigorous workout, it should beat at a rate of 119 (.70 x 170) to 144 (.85 x 170).

Finding the beat

You can check your pulse either on the underside of your wrist or in your neck between the windpipe and the large neck muscles. Feeling your pulse can take some practice. Use the tips of your index and middle fingers, and don't press too hard. Count the number of beats for 10 seconds (you'll need a watch with a second hand, of course); then multiply the total by six. That number will tell you how hard your heart is beating and whether a workout is meeting your intensity goal.

The talk test

Does all this math sound too complicated? Don't despair. There are simpler, albeit less scientific, ways to determine whether your workouts are doing your heart some good. If you work up a sweat and feel slightly out of breath for about 15 minutes after your workout, you're probably going at a good, heart-healthy pace. You can also try the "talk test." If you can carry on a conversation

Heart Math: How Hard Should You Work?

Age	Maximum Heart Rate	50% to 70% of Maximum	70% to 85% of Maximum
25	195	97 to 136	136 to 165
30	190	95 to 133	133 to 161
35	185	92 to 129	129 to 157
40	180	90 to 126	126 to 153
45	175	87 to 122	122 to 148
50	170	85 to 119	119 to 144
55	165	82 to 115	115 to 140
60	160	80 to 112	112 to 136
65	155	77 to 108	108 to 131
70	150	75 to 105	105 to 127
75	145	72 to 101	101 to 123
80	140	70 to 98	98 to 119

with an exercise partner—or sing out loud to yourself—with only a slight effort, then you are probably within your target range. On the other hand, if you find yourself huffing and puffing too much to talk properly, then slow down! You're working too hard.

How long?

Once you reach your target intensity during a workout, you want to stay there long enough for your cardiovascular system to reap the benefits. At a minimum, you should try to exercise for 30 minutes within your target pulse range. (Warm-up and cool-down time does not count because during those parts of the workout your pulse drops below the target range.)

Of course, if you want to gradually expand your aerobic workout to 45 or 60 minutes, or even longer, your blood pressure will thank you for it. Long, continuous workouts are helpful for losing weight because the body tends to start burning significant amounts of fat only after 30 minutes of vigorous activity.

Go short, go long? During the last decade, experts at the Centers for Disease Control and Prevention (CDC) and elsewhere have offered good news to people who seem allergic to the thought of donning gym shorts, a tee shirt, and other exercise gear. Pointing to several studies, the CDC officials have declared that a workout doesn't have to last for 30 continuous minutes to help your heart. You can, instead, divide those 30 minutes into shorter bouts of activity over the course of a day—a quick 10-minute stint on your home stationary bike in the morning, for example, followed later in the day by a brisk 20-minute walk. Furthermore, according to the CDC, ordinary activities—such as washing the car, vacuuming the house, and gardening—"count" as heart-healthy activities.

Not all researchers agree with the CDC on this "exercise lite" advice, however. Some say there is no good scientific evidence to back up the claim that intermittent bursts of exercise are as good for health as a solid half-hour workout. Still, everyone agrees that almost any physical activity is better than none at all. So on those days when you don't have a long stretch of time to devote to exercise, take

Ciao to Calories

If losing weight is one of your exercise goals, then you may want to keep track of your calorie burn during your workouts. The precise number of calories you expend during a particular activity depends on your body weight. The more you weigh, the more calories you burn.

Activity	Calories burned every 30 minutes if you weigh...			
	125 lb.	150 lb.	175 lb.	200 lb.
Bicycling (6 mph)	102	120	138	156
Bicycling (12 mph)	178	210	241	273
Cross-country skiing	297	350	402	455
Jumping rope	318	375	431	487
Running (5½ mph)	314	370	425	481
Running (7 mph)	391	460	529	598
Swimming (25 yd./min)	119	140	161	182
Swimming (50 yd./min)	212	250	287	325
Tennis (singles)	170	200	230	260
Walking (2 mph)	102	120	138	156
Walking (3 mph)	136	160	184	208
Walking (4 mph)	187	220	253	286

several short "health" breaks. Walk your dog or rake the leaves. Or turn on the radio and dance! Just get moving.

How often?

You now know how intense your aerobic workout should be (at least 50 percent of your maximum heart rate) and for how long (at least 30 minutes). The final big question is: How often should you exercise? Most experts recommend three to five times a week. Anything less and your blood pressure is unlikely to improve; anything more and you risk injuring your muscles without significantly improving your cardiovascular system.

To avoid injury, especially if you're overweight or have been inactive for a while, space out your aerobic workouts over a week. Your body will thank you for the days off! Rest days shouldn't be "no movement at all" days, however. You can still go for a leisurely walk, or poke around in the garden, or maybe even play a round of golf or splash about in the pool. You just don't have to pay attention to the intensity or length of the workout.

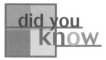

An Aerobic Smorgasbord

To find the exerciser within, choose an activity that is not only going to make you sweat but also give you a sense of accomplishment and—dare we say—joy. And then learn to be your own yardstick, finding happiness in your personal progress rather than homing in on your best friend's greater accomplishments.

Walking. This is the easiest, least expensive, and safest aerobic activity. It requires no special equipment—except comfortable shoes—and can be done just about anywhere. You can walk alone or with friends, outdoors or indoors (on a treadmill or through a mall). If you've been sedentary, start slowly—maybe with a 5- or 10-minute stroll—and then gradually increase both speed and distance.

Tip: Strike the ground first with your heel, then with the ball of your foot, and finally push off with your toes. This sequence will help prevent shin splints and shin pain. Not surprisingly, good walking shoes will have extra cushioning in the heel area, the site of greatest impact.

Running. This activity tunes up your cardiovascular system quickly, with much less of a time investment than walking. Thus, it can be a good activity for busy people. The only equipment you'll need is a high-quality pair of running shoes. Start slowly—and only after you can walk two miles at a brisk pace. Running can be hard on the knees. If you've suffered from any knee problems, talk with your doctor before starting a running program. Or consider walking, swimming, or biking.

Tip: Good shoes are a must. Intensity and balance are a concern for pregnant women, older people, and the obese. Also, to protect your joints, crouch (like Groucho Marx) when you're running downhill.

Bicycling. A great aerobic activity for beginners, bicycling enables you to build up your endurance slowly and with minimal stress on your leg joints. It can be done outdoors (preferably on some kind of bike path) or indoors on a stationary bike. Either way, you'll need a good, sturdy bike—as well as a helmet if you're riding outdoors. By the way, as it turns out, pedaling rapidly in an "easy" gear gives you the best aerobic workout.

Exercise without Walls

If you are the independent type who feels confined by the parameters of a program or the commitment to a highly demanding sport, here is a great way to burn 2,000 calories a week without running a marathon or participating in super-structured activities:

Situation	Activity	Calories per Week
On the job or at home	Climbing two flights of stairs daily	300
	Walking 1 to 2 miles a day on the job	750
Leisure walking	1 to 2 hours or 5 miles/week	350
Moderate sports like golf, tennis, or swimming	2 hours per week	750

Tip: Pay attention to your seat height. Position the seat so that when you extend one leg fully on the down pedal, with your foot flat, your knee is slightly bent. If the seat is too low, you'll stress your knees. If it's too high, you'll place undue force on your back. Also, adjust the handlebar's stem height so it's 2 to 5 centimeters below the tip of the seat.

Rope jumping. Borrow a trick from world-class boxers to build up your heart and lungs: Jump rope. Although rope jumping won't raise your heart rate as consistently as running, this is still a top-notch aerobic activity. It takes coordination and practice, however, as well as plenty of room in which to twirl the rope. Rope jumping can quickly elevate your heart rate to training levels. So start slowly, perhaps by alternating rope jumping with walking.

Tip: Avoid jumping on asphalt or other hard surfaces (try a surface with give—a wood floor, carpet, or an exercise mat) and be sure to wear cushioned shoes; rope jumping can be hard on the knees. Also, purchase a beaded rope, which won't tangle.

Swimming. Because it doesn't stress bones, joints, or muscles, swimming is an excellent aerobic activity, particularly for people who are overweight or those who have arthritis or other joint problems.

Tip: Take a few swimming lessons if you haven't done so recently. Some new techniques—specifically the S-patterned stroke—help prevent shoulder problems and allow you to swim more efficiently.

Skating. Whether you do it on ice or on asphalt, skating can be a great aerobic conditioner. Be sure to keep a vigorous and steady pace for 30 minutes. Skating requires special equipment, of course, and special skills.

Stair climbing. This easy-to-do activity helps the heart with minimal wear and tear on the ankles and knees. Of course, we're talking stair-climbing machines here, not actual stairs. Using stairs instead of the elevator is a good idea for "mini" workouts, but most people would find it hard, if not impossible, to do a full 30-minute aerobic workout in a stairwell.

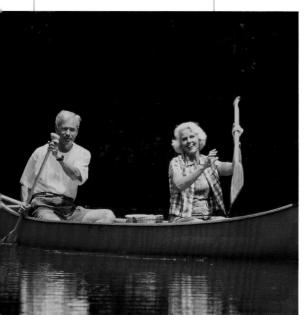

Tip: Avoid overstressing your knees on a stair-climbing machine by making sure that your extended leg is slightly bent and both knees are aligned behind your toes.

Rowing. This activity offers superb cardiovascular conditioning. If a rowing club is located in your area and you can afford the fees, you may want to consider signing up for classes and perhaps even joining a team. Most people who row for exercise, however, do so on machines that simulate the open-water experience. Machines that have a flywheel and chain drive are usually the easiest and most effective models to use.

Tip: Avoid the common mistake of sliding your seat backward before you move your arms. Instead, slide back and pull at the same time. To protect your joints, never lock your knees or elbows while rowing.

Watch Out! Safer Aerobic Sessions

- ◗ Warm up. For best results, start each exercise session—whether it be a swim in the pool or a jog in the park—with a warmup of 5 to 10 minutes of moderate aerobic activity that heats up your muscles, making them more pliable and less likely to tear. Walk at a moderate pace, ride on an exercise bike, or even march in place.

- ◗ Dress for success. Choose clothes that allow free movement. Stretchy materials and elastic waistbands are ideal. Avoid cotton, which absorbs sweat, leaving you feeling clammy.

- ◗ Foot joy. Certain sports do require specific kinds of footwear. Don't start running in walking shoes or wear running shoes to an aerobics class (you may have trouble doing side-to-side steps and may raise your risk for ankle sprains). Make sure to match your shoe to your main activity.

○ Drink deep. Staying hydrated can prevent dizziness, cramps, exhaustion, and even collapse. Drink a tall glass of water at least 20 minutes before your workout, and as you exercise, sip from a water bottle—about two ounces at least every 10 minutes.

○ Cool down. End every session with a cooldown (about half as long as your warmup) during which you gradually reduce the intensity of your exercise. Follow the cooldown with some stretches designed to loosen up the muscles you've exercised.

○ Take baby steps. Many people start out full-throttle—and end up injured or burned out. Instead, think small and build on your successes.

Weighing In on Weight Training

Doctors used to discourage people with high blood pressure from engaging in strength training, fearing that it would trigger a sudden spike in blood pressure. Now, however, they're rethinking that advice. A recent review of four decades of research suggests that building muscle may actually lower blood pressure.

In fact, the American Heart Association now recommends that people with and without heart disease include weight training in their regular exercise routine (people with heart disease, however, should check with their doctor first).

A Strong Case for Strength

From lifting laundry or a child or grandchild to lugging heavy files and a computer home from the office, many of our daily activities require muscles that can handle the load. To keep our muscles fit and strong, however, we need to use them—regularly, consistently. Yet few of us do, which is why we tend to lose an average of 3 to 5 percent of our muscle tissue during each decade of our adult lives. No wonder we find it increasingly difficult to perform once-routine tasks, like carrying groceries or shoveling snow. Weaker muscles can also lead to joint stiffness and fatigue, causing us to feel older faster.

Proving your metal. But all is not doom and gloom. Not only does weight training prevent muscle loss but it also can reverse it. And here's the really good news: It is never too late to rebuild your muscles. You can do it at any age, even if you've

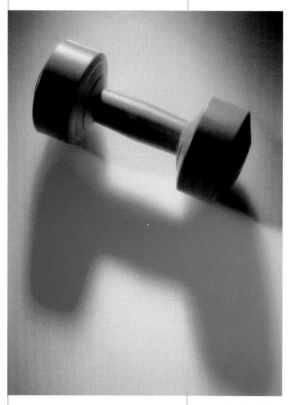

never done any kind of strength training before. One study that included several hundred nursing-home residents aged 72 to 98 found that just 10 weeks of weight training more than doubled the participants' strength. As a result, they were able to walk longer distances and climb stairs more easily than before their stint with weights.

Stronger muscles are not the only reason why you should take up weight training, however. As you lose muscle, you burn fewer calories, upping your risk for becoming overweight—not a very good thing for maintaining normal BP levels.

Building lean muscle mass not only burns calories while you are doing it and right afterward—some studies show that your metabolism remains elevated for up to 48 hours after lifting—but also does so by increasing your basal metabolism. Muscle is much more metabolically active than fat and, as a result, burns more calories than its flabby opposite—even while you are resting in your easy chair or bed.

> **Pressure Point:** Strength training does more than build muscle. Studies show that it may also reduce levels of artery-clogging LDL cholesterol.

Muscle also beefs up bones, which need stimulation from muscle to stay strong and to become denser. So gaining strength will also help you gain the upper hand on osteoporosis, the bone-thinning (and often permanently disabling) disease that can lead to fractures later in life.

Lift Your Load

Contrary to stereotypes on television and in the movies, weight training doesn't have to consist of heaving a huge, weighted barbell over your head while your eyes bulge out. That kind of Popeye-like activity is sure to send your blood pressure up—way up—not down. In fact, Olympic weight lifters have been known to drive up their BP to 480/320. Instead of hoisting the greatest amount of weight you can, your goal in weight training is to lift relatively lighter loads in succession. Think endurance, not bulk.

Most gyms and health clubs offer a "circuit" of special weight-training machines (sometimes called weight-resistance machines) that, despite their daunting size and elaborate workings, are easy and safe to use. This equipment enables you to focus on strengthening one isolated muscle group at a time. To get the most out of the machines, have a fitness trainer instruct you on their use.

Home bodies. If you are the stay-at-home type, you can accomplish as much on your living room rug with a few light dumbbells (sold at almost every sports-equipment store) and a good instructional book. Start with a two-and-a-half-pound set, then work your way up to heavier ones. This is aptly called progressive resistance: After your muscles adjust to the load you have been lifting, you increase the load again in order to move to the next strength level. (See *Make a Muscle: A Beginner's Strength Program,* pages 124-129.)

Eventually, you might want to graduate to a barbell with weighted plates and perhaps a bench. Be sure to follow the manufacturer's instructions on how to set up and safely use the equipment. You might even want to hire a qualified training expert to come into your home once or twice to demonstrate correct technique and form.

A simple solution. You can, of course, strengthen your muscles without any special equipment at all. A couple of soup cans or two half-gallon milk jugs filled with sand can take the

> **CAUTION**
>
> Weight training is okay as long as you have your high blood pressure under control. Don't lift weights if you have a systolic blood pressure of 160 mm Hg or higher or a diastolic blood pressure of 100 mm Hg or higher.

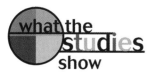

place of dumbbells. Or use your own body weight to build up strength. Simple exercises like pushups, pullups, leg lifts, and abdominal crunches can help you develop strong muscles.

When Will You See a Change?

Your body contours should change within a month of consistent weight training. (If not, check with a pro for some corrections.) Don't expect big results, though—that will take three to six months of steady work. Some muscles grow stronger much faster than others; in general, large muscles like the chest, back, and buttocks develop first. Don't worry about bulking up too much. It takes hours of work per day to build huge muscles.

Watch Out! Safer Strength Training

❍ Warm up your muscles and prevent injury by doing 5 to 10 minutes of gentle aerobic exercise before each weight-training session. Any kind of aerobics will do: Walk in place, jump rope, or ride a stationary bike.

❍ Maintain a slow and steady pace. Always begin with light weights and lift in a slow, controlled manner.

❍ Maintain good form. Follow the instructions for technique and repetitions taught to you by your trainer or described in your workout book.

❍ Breathe out while lifting a weight; breathe in while lowering it.

❍ Train both sides of your body equally. Use the same amount of weights in your left and right hands, even if one side of your body seems stronger.

❍ Give your muscles a break. Don't exercise the same muscle groups two days in a row.

❍ To avoid stiffness and injury, be sure to stretch your muscles when your strength-training session is over.

Make a Muscle: A Beginner's Strength Program

Here is a simple strength-training program of 14 exercises to get you started. Do two to three sets of 10 to 12 repetitions of each exercise, unless stated otherwise.

Lower Body

Adduction

1 Lie on your right side with your left leg angled in front of you and the inside of your left foot resting on the floor. Keep your right leg straight without locking your knee.

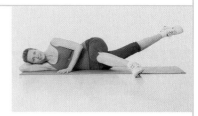

2 Raise your right (lower) leg as high as you comfortably can. Hold for one second, then slowly lower it to within one inch of the floor. Hold, then repeat. Your lower leg should not touch the floor until the end of the set.

3 After each set, switch sides.

To step up the exercise, add ankle weights to the leg you're lifting. If you have knee problems, place the weights above your knee.

Abduction

1 Lie on your right side with your right knee and hip each bent at a 45-degree angle. Keep your upper leg nearly straight, and keep your torso straight to avoid stressing your lower back.

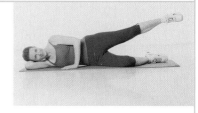

2 Raise your upper leg as high as you comfortably can. Hold for one second, then slowly lower it until it is almost touching your lower leg. Your upper leg should not touch your lower leg until the end of the set.

3 After each set, switch sides.

Squats

1 Stand in front of a chair with your feet about hip-width apart. Keep your body erect and your chin raised slightly throughout this exercise.

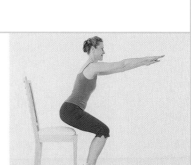

2 Slowly lower your hips toward the chair as if you're about to sit. Just before your body touches it, return to a standing position. Keep your back straight, your knees behind your toes, your weight centered over your midfoot and heels (not over your toes), and your feet flat on the floor.

Lunges

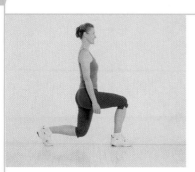

1. Start with your feet hip-width apart or slightly closer. Raise your chin slightly throughout this exercise.

2. Take a large step forward with your right leg, planting your foot firmly on the floor with your toes pointed forward or slightly inward. Align your right knee over your right foot. Keep your back straight and your knee behind the toes of your forward foot.

3. Bring your left knee straight down until it is an inch or two from the floor. To raise yourself, press firmly into the floor with your right foot while extending your right knee.

4. Return to the initial standing position and repeat with your left leg forward.

Upper Body

Chest Press

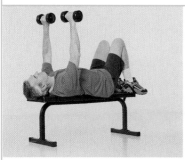

1. Lie faceup on a bench. Keep your feet on the bench, knees bent, to support your lower back. Hold a pair of dumbbells at your chest, your palms facing your knees.

2. Exhale as you press the weights upward, bringing them close together but not touching, and extending your elbows almost fully.

3. Inhale as you lower the weights slowly, reversing the movement. Lower your elbows to just below torso level.

One-Arm Dumbbell Row

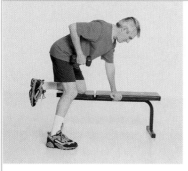

1. Rest your left knee and hand on the edge of a bench or firm chair or sofa. Bend your right knee slightly so your weight is distributed evenly on both legs. Lightly grasp a dumbbell with your right hand, and let it hang straight down by your side. Keep your working arm close to your body, your back straight, and your shoulders level.

2. Exhale as you pull the dumbbell upward toward your waist, stopping when it almost touches your torso.

3. Inhale as you lower it slowly to the original position. Switch sides at the end of each set.

Kickback

1. Rest your right knee and right hand on a bench or chair and extend your left leg behind you, with your left foot flat on the floor. Grasp a dumbbell lightly in your left hand, keeping your elbow at your side, your arm bent at a 45-degree angle.

2. Exhale as you straighten your left arm almost fully. Keep your elbow at your side and move only your forearm.

3. Pause, then inhale as you lower your arm to its original 45-degree angle. After each set, switch sides and work your other arm.

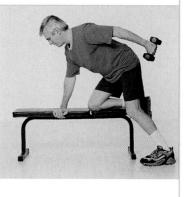

Seated Biceps Curl

1. Lightly grasp a pair of dumbbells, keeping your arms straight at your sides, your palms facing forward.

2. Exhale as you raise the weights toward your shoulders, pinning your elbows at your sides so that only your forearms move. Also make sure to tense your abdominal muscles for support.

3. Inhale as you lower your arms and weights slowly back to the original position.

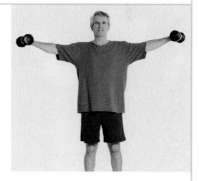

Standing Lateral Raise

1. You can sit or stand for this exercise. Lightly grasp a pair of dumbbells and let them hang down at your sides while bending your elbows slightly. Tense your abdominal muscles for support during this exercise.

2. Exhale as you raise your arms outward until they are parallel to the floor. Your wrists, elbows, and shoulders should be in a straight line. Don't lock elbows.

3. Inhale as you lower your arms and weights until they nearly touch your sides.

Midsection

Strong muscles in your core—your torso—stabilize your body, allowing you to sit for long stretches without slumping or to rake leaves (your arms move while your trunk provides leverage). Strong abdominal and back muscles help prevent back strains and also help power your golf swing and your swimming stroke.

Reverse Crunch

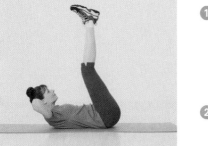

1. Lie faceup on a mat or carpet with your knees bent. Raise one leg at a time, straightening each leg so that the soles of your feet face the ceiling. Raise your head from the floor slightly, placing your palms loosely behind your head to provide neck support.

2. As you exhale, contract your abdominal muscles (abs) to pull back your legs about 30 degrees toward your head. Be sure to use your abs, not your leg muscles, to accomplish this movement.

3. Inhale as you relax your abs to slowly return your legs to their original position.

4. Do two sets of 15 reps.

Oblique Twist

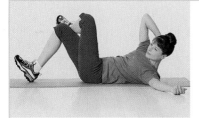

1. Lie faceup on a mat or carpet with your knees bent. Place your left ankle across your right knee and your left hand palm up on the floor perpendicular to your body. Place your right palm behind your head to provide neck support.

2. Exhale as you raise your upper body, bringing your right shoulder toward your left knee.

3. Pause briefly, then inhale as you slowly lower your upper body to the mat. Your right hand should not pull your head forward. Switch sides.

4. Do two sets of 15 reps, each side.

Crunch

1. Lie faceup on a mat or carpet with your knees bent and your feet on the floor. Point your toes up to provide extra back support. Place both hands under your head with the index fingers and thumbs of each hand touching. Throughout the exercise, be sure your lower back is pressed into the floor and always avoid any bouncing or jerking movements.

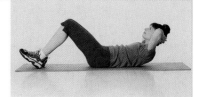

2. As you exhale, curl your upper body toward your thighs about 30 degrees. Pause briefly, then inhale as you slowly lower yourself.

3. Do two sets of 15 reps each.

Expert Tip

When working any muscle group, exercise your larger muscles first. If you work your small muscles first, they'll be too tired to support your larger muscles during their workout. Using this strategy, do your abdominal exercises in this order: Reverse Crunch, Oblique Twist, Crunch.

Lower Extension

1. Lie facedown on a mat with your arms resting comfortably at your sides.

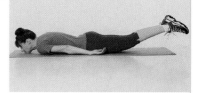

2. As you exhale, keep your upper body in contact with the mat and gently raise your legs upward as high as you comfortably can. Inhale as you lower your legs toward the floor.

3. Start with a goal of one set of 10 to 15 reps.

Upper Extension

1. Lie facedown on a mat with your arms resting at your sides.

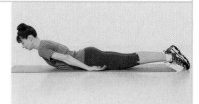

2. Exhale as you gently raise your upper body slowly off the floor as high as you comfortably can.

3. Inhale as you lower yourself toward the floor. Allow your chest to tap the floor momentarily between each rep.

4. Start with a goal of one set of 10 to 15 reps.

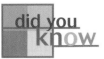

did you know

▶ *In 1998, the American College of Sports Medicine expanded the traditional goals of exercise— developing aerobic fitness and muscle strength—to include a third key goal: flexibility. The college urged all Americans to add stretching to their regular exercise program, based on the "growing evidence of its multiple benefits."*

Stretching: Flexible Benefits

The average adult's flexibility declines by about 5 percent per decade. Not a good thing. Not only does flexibility prevent your muscles and joints from getting stiff (a real problem as we get older) but it also lowers your risk of injuring yourself during your aerobic and weight-training workouts.

What's more, flexibility exercises can also release stress-related tension, which may help lower your blood pressure. Beyond that, stretching is a needed counterpoint to strength training. When you strength-train, your muscles tend to shorten, which makes you less flexible. Regular stretching will elongate those muscles, reduce any soreness, lower your injury risk, and provide you with a greater range of motion. Stretching also improves coordination and workout performance and may lessen recovery time between workouts. Stretching rids muscles of lactic acid and other waste products that build up in the muscles when you exercise them.

The idea behind stretching is simple: When a muscle is pulled slightly beyond its normal length, it gradually adapts to its longer length and increases a joint's range of motion. Try to do at least 15 minutes of stretching—or flexibility exercises—every day. The best time to stretch is during or after a workout, when your muscles are warmed up. Don't flex before you get your muscles moving; when you stretch taut, cold muscles, you risk injury. A warm swimming pool is an ideal place to stretch: Your limbs are supported and the warm temperature limbers up muscles.

Stretch and strengthen. The benefits of stretching go beyond preventing injury to muscles; the activity could actually help build additional strength. A new study shows that strength trainers who stretched after each exercise were nearly 20 percent stronger after 10 weeks than those who didn't limber up between moves. "Stretching makes muscles more receptive to strength building—probably because by contracting the muscles through weight training, then lengthening them with stretching, you're maximizing their potential," says Wayne Westcott, Ph.D., director of fitness research at the South Shore YMCA in Quincy, Massachusetts, who conducted the study.

> **Pressure Point:** On days when you don't work out, do your stretching in the evening, before you go to bed. Not only will it soothe your muscles but it will also calm your mind and help you sleep.

A major selling point of stretching is that you don't need special clothing, equipment, or an opening in your social calendar to do it. You can do it at work, in your car, while watching TV in your living room. So in many ways, it is a less stressful endeavor than preparing to take a walk or lifting weights in a gym. In fact, advocates of stretching suggest that you will be benefitting more than your muscles if you stretch regularly. It dissipates tension and stress—elevators to your blood pressure—and helps align the body, easing areas of compression that may impede the workings of the body's organs.

CAUTION

Avoid "bounce" stretching—repeated, brief, forceful stretches. They can actually cause damage and increase stiffness.

Stretching exercises come in many forms, but those derived from hatha yoga are among the most effective. You can begin by taking a yoga class or by following the instructions offered in a yoga video or book. You can also try out the simple stretching program on the next three pages.

Watch Out! Safer Stretching

- You should never stretch a cold muscle; it is always wise to warm up first. Do your stretching at the end of your exercise routine; or warm up muscles with a slow walk or with a 5- or 10-minute stint on the treadmill—then stretch.

- Ease into a stretch to the point where you begin to feel mild discomfort—never beyond—and then hold that "maximum" position for 10 to 30 seconds.

- Don't hold your breath while stretching. Your muscles need the oxygen. Exhale as you try to stretch farther.

- Form is everything. Don't cheat your stretch by contorting your body or using other joints to compensate for inflexibility.

- Stop if you feel any pain. Pain indicates you are damaging tissues. You should feel the stretch, not pain.

Flex Time: A Beginner's Stretching Program

All the stretches that follow are particularly effective when combined with the strength-building exercises on the previous pages. Once you've fully extended a muscle, hold the stretch for a few seconds—never bounce. Stretch only after warming up to avoid damaging both muscles and tendons.

Lower Body

These stretches are especially important if you spend a lot of time sitting. Perform each one four or more times.

Quad Stretch

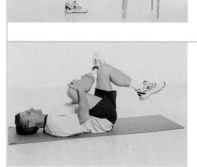

1. With your left hand on a chair back for balance, bend your right knee and grasp your ankle with your right hand.

2. Pull slightly, producing a strong stretch across the front of your thigh. Hold two to four seconds.

3. Switch legs and repeat.

Across-the-Knee Raise

1. Lie on your back with both knees bent and your feet flat on the floor, your arms out to your sides. Place your right ankle across your left knee.

2. Exhale as your bring your left leg toward your chest, carrying your right ankle with it. If needed, use your arms for support. Hold the stretch two to four seconds.

3. Switch legs and repeat.

Straight-Leg Stretch

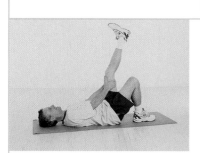

1. Lie on your back, both knees bent, and feet flat on the floor. Extend your left leg upward until nearly straight.

2. With both hands behind your thigh, exhale, pulling your leg gently toward your chest to feel the stretch in your hamstring. Hold two to four seconds.

3. Switch legs and repeat.

Upper Body

Behind-the-Back Stretch

1. While standing or sitting, bend your right elbow, grasp it with your left hand, and reach your right hand down toward your left shoulder blade.

2. Pull on your right elbow slightly until you feel a stretch along the back of your upper arm. There is very little range of motion with this exercise. After two or three reps, switch arms and repeat.

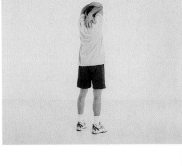

Straight-Arm Extension

1. While standing, fully extend your left arm so your palm is facing forward. Grasp it with your right hand.

2. Exhale as you press gently against that palm, bending your wrist back until you feel a stretch across the inside of your left elbow. Hold, then release. There is very little range of motion with this exercise. Perform two or three reps, then repeat with your right arm.

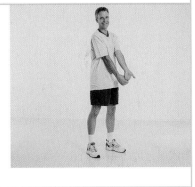

Hand-on-Wall Stretch

1. Stretch your left arm behind you, palm against a wall, elbow slightly bent.

2. Exhale as you turn slowly to the right, maintaining the bend in your elbow, until you feel a stretch across your left shoulder and chest. Hold, then release. Repeat several times, then switch arms.

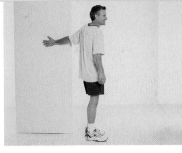

Extended-Arm Pull

1. Stand or sit with your arms extended in front of you. Grasp your left wrist with your right hand.

2. Pull your left arm to the right, across your chest. Hold and release. Repeat with your right arm.

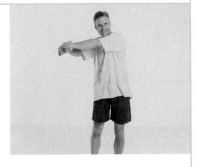

Core Body

Knee Hug

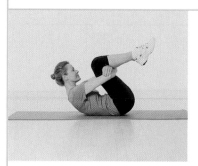

1. Lie on your back with your knees bent, feet flat on the floor.

2. Exhale as you use your abs and hips to pull your knees toward your chest. Place your arms behind your knees with your palms on your elbows. Use your arms to pull your knees closer to your chest.

3. Hold for two or three seconds, release your legs, lowering your feet slowly to the floor. Repeat.

Press-Ups

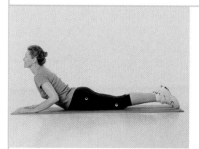

1. Lie facedown on the floor with your hands near your shoulders, palms against the floor.

2. Exhale as you straighten your arms to raise your upper body, keeping your elbows tucked close to your sides. Keep your hips and lower body relaxed and on the floor.

3. Stop when you begin to feel a stretch in your lower back or waist. Hold for two seconds before lowering yourself to the original position. Repeat.

Side Twist

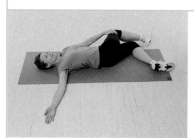

1. Lie on your back, your arms out to the sides, your knees bent, and your feet flat on the floor.

2. Exhale as you lower both legs to the left, keeping your knees together and bent. With your left hand, gently press down on your right leg until you feel a strong stretch along your right side. Repeat two to four reps; switch sides.

Cat's Back

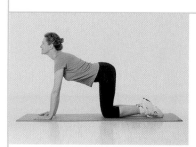

1. Rest on your hands and knees, keeping your back flat.

2. Exhale as you curl your back upward and lower your head until you're looking at your abdomen. Hold for a moment.

3. Inhale as you lower your back slowly until it is arched as far as is comfortable, raising your head so you're looking up toward the ceiling. Repeat.

The Flabby Truth

Now that you know the activity formula for helping to lower blood pressure, you need to ask yourself a question: How much exercise do you really get? Be honest. Dashing to the refrigerator during a TV commercial break is not an aerobic activity—unless, of course, you have a very big house.

Studies show that most of us grossly overestimate how much physical activity we do in our day-to-day lives. We like to think that we're active beavers, but in reality most of us are sedentary slugs. Few of us have jobs that require vigorous physical activity; nor do many of us get up and flex our muscles much during our leisure time. We spend a lot of time sitting on our ever-expanding haunches—at desks, behind the wheel of our cars, in front of our television and computer screens. And when confronted with the option of using some of our flabby muscles—such as walking up a flight of stairs rather than taking an elevator—we almost always pass…When was the last time you were in a stairwell of a building with elevators?

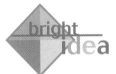

For a realistic appraisal of exactly how much physical activity you get, wear a pedometer—a device that records distances walked—for a few days. You may be surprised by what you learn. One nurse who was sure she walked five or six miles each day on her job donned a pedometer as an experiment. She soon discovered (much to her amazement) that she actually walked only about a mile a day.

Watch Out! Ask the Doctor

Many people can rev up their physical activity without seeing a doctor. But if you take high blood pressure medication, have heart disease, have suffered a heart attack or stroke, or have another serious health problem, you should check with your doctor before starting or increasing an exercise program.

Take a Baby Step

You acknowledge that you tend to be a slug when it comes to moving your muscles. You also recognize that regular exercise would not only help you lower your blood pressure but also improve other aspects of both your physical and emotional health. But how can you shoehorn an exercise program—one that includes aerobic, weight training, and flexibility exercises, for goodness sake—into your impossibly hectic schedule?

Don't panic, and definitely don't give up. You can develop a personalized exercise program that works.

Working in a Workout

If a full-blown exercise program sounds daunting, channel these "baby steps" of increased activity into your life.

- Play ball with your kids or grandchildren.

- Cancel your newspaper delivery and walk to the store every morning to buy it instead.

- Take out your dog for an extra walk every day, or change your route to cover hillier terrain.

- Dust off your bicycle and take it for a weekend spin through the neighborhood.

- Take two extra full turns around the mall whenever you go shopping.

- Choose the farthest parking spot and let your legs do the walking.

- Walk the golf course rather than taking a cart.

- Rake leaves by hand instead of using a blower.

- Stretch and strengthen your ankles and lower-leg muscles while you watch TV. First, alternately flex and extend your feet. Then make circles in the air with your feet, rotating your ankles clockwise, then counterclockwise.

> **Aerobics.** You need to find three to five 30-minute slots of time, preferably on alternating days, to do your aerobic workouts. Remember to give yourself warmup and cooldown time on either side of that 30 minutes.

> **Weight training.** Aim for 15 to 30 minutes of weight training two times a week on nonconsecutive days. To make things simple, schedule weight training on the days you don't do aerobics. Again, make sure you allow yourself some warmup and cooldown time.

>**Flexibility exercises.** About 15 minutes of daily stretching should be your goal. You can fit this in as part of your cooldown period after workouts. Or you can set aside 15 minutes during your day for flexing your muscles, either in one single chunk of time (before bedtime is best) or in a series of "mini-stretches" throughout the day.

Now plug those commitments into the chart below:

Day	Aerobic Workout	Weight Training	Flexibility Exercises
Monday	Time:	Time:	Time:
Tuesday	Time:	Time:	Time:
Wednesday	Time:	Time:	Time:
Thursday	Time:	Time:	Time:
Friday	Time:	Time:	Time:
Saturday	Time:	Time:	Time:
Sunday	Time:	Time:	Time:

Treat these commitments as mandatory appointments—ones you will not break except under exceptional circumstances. If you've scheduled a 30-minute walk at noon, for example, don't let a friend persuade you to meet her for lunch instead. If you've set aside a half hour right after work for weight training, don't get sidetracked by a telephone call. Persistence is the key to starting and maintaining a successful exercise program. You need to make exercise an integral part of your daily routine—as automatic as brushing your teeth or taking a shower.

The Tortoise Factor: Slow and Steady

A lifetime of inactivity isn't something you should abandon in a flash. If you are a veteran of the couch potato wars and are 30 pounds or more overweight to boot, you don't want to rush right out and attempt to run a mile or to do 50 ab crunches. The easiest path to exercise burnout—not to mention injuries—is to push your body too hard too fast.

Get a goal. Begin by knowing what you want to accomplish. Set reasonable but specific long-term health goals. If you have high blood pressure, for example, you may want to establish a

Problem—Solution: Getting Over Those Exercise Hurdles

Barrier	Possible Solution
You lack motivation or confidence. *"I can't do this."*	• Exercise with a friend. Or join an exercise class or group (like a walking or running club). • Keep an exercise journal. Record and celebrate your progress. • Devise ways you can inexpensively reward yourself when you meet one of your exercise goals. Then do it!
You lack time. *"I'm too busy today."* *"Something more important has come up."*	• Sit down at the beginning of the week and make exercise "appointments" with yourself. Treat those appointments seriously. • Let your friends and relatives know how important your exercise schedule is to you and your health. Ask for their support. (Or invite them to join you!) • On days when you simply don't have a long block of time to exercise, aim for small 10- to 15-minute activity sessions.
You lack access to exercise facilities or equipment. *"I don't have the right shoes."* *"I can't afford to join a gym."* *"It's too cold outside."*	• Walking is an excellent aerobic exercise. It can be done almost anywhere and with no special equipment except a comfortable pair of shoes. • Weight training and stretching can also be done at home without any special equipment. • Use exercise videos on those days when the weather is unsuitable for outdoor activities.
You had a previous negative experience trying to start an exercise program. *"I don't like to exercise." "I'm no good at it."*	• Start slowly with a low-intensity exercise, like walking. • Try to identify the source of your negative attitude toward exercise. Work through it. • Join an exercise support group, or exercise with friends.
You're overweight. *"I'm too fat." "I'm too out-of-shape."*	• Start slowly with a low-intensity aerobic exercise, like walking. Biking and water aerobics are also good for large bodies. • Be aware that exercise becomes easier over time.
You're worried that exercising may harm your health or cause you to injure yourself. *"I'm so out-of-shape, I'll have a heart attack or stroke if I start exercising." "I have bad knees." "I'm too old."*	• Check with your doctor before getting started. • Begin slowly with a low-intensity exercise, such as walking. • To limit injuries, vary the types of activities you do. You'll also have more fun! • Join an exercise class specially designed for people your age.
You experience discomfort or pain while exercising. *"Exercising hurts." "I always injure myself."*	• Talk with your doctor about what might have caused the pain. • Exercise with less intensity. Be sure to take days off between strenuous workouts. • Switch to exercises that put less stress on joints—biking, swimming, or water aerobics, for example.

six-month goal of lowering your systolic blood pressure by 4 mm Hg and your diastolic blood pressure by 2 mm Hg. You may also want to lose 10 pounds within that same time frame.

Once you know what your long-term goals are, you can set some specific exercise goals to reach them. But start slowly. Remember: You didn't get out of shape overnight, so don't expect to get into shape overnight either. If your aerobics goal is to run for 30 minutes three times a week, for example, spend several weeks walking before you even think about picking up the pace. Once you can walk briskly for 30 minutes with ease, then—and only then—should you introduce running into your workout. Try a one-minute jog every five minutes or so within your walk. Then gradually increase the jogging time and decrease the walking time. (Be sure to always start with a warm-up walk and end with some stretching.)

> **Pressure Point:** Exercise tends to lower your blood pressure the most during the first five hours after your workout.

Some pain, some gain. Expect some stiffness and soreness at first. After all, you may be asking your muscles to move in ways they haven't done so in years! Over time, the workouts should become easier, however, and you'll begin to notice yourself getting stronger, more energetic, and perhaps even leaner. You'll also start to accomplish some of your health goals—at which point you'll want to set new ones. Good health—and lower blood pressure—requires a lifetime commitment.

No-Excuse Exercising

All of us have our favorite excuses for not exercising. It's very likely that you recognize one (or all) of the following perennials: "I'm too busy." "I don't have the right equipment." "I'm too fat."

It's important to recognize the excuses and other barriers that are likely to get in your way as you try to start—and stick with!—an exercise program. As soon as you hit one of these barriers (and we all do from time to time), step back for a moment, evaluate the situation, and look for a creative solution. The chart on the facing page, offers sensible counterpoints to your most creative excuses.

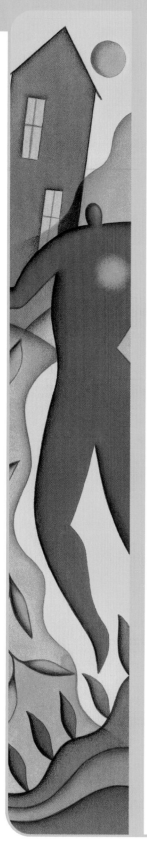

Walking Away from High Blood Pressure

Exercise is not Carolyn Johnson's cup of tea. "Well, no, I'm not particularly thrilled about it," says Johnson, 70, of Prescott, Arizona. "But it sure beats taking pills for a lifetime."

Johnson is referring to pills for high blood pressure. Three years ago, she noticed spells of "anxiety and heaviness, like some weight was on me," she says. The feelings were linked to her blood pressure, which soared to 156/74 mm Hg.

Because her hypertension only occurred episodically, Johnson's doctor was willing to try managing the disease without medication. "I'm not a happy pilltaker," she says.

She's not a happy exerciser, either. Johnson's doctor recommended diet changes and exercise. The less-salt diet she could live with, but the more-exercise program was another story. Although her daughters were faithful exercisers, Johnson grew up in an era when joggers were few and far between and probably had too much time on their hands, anyway. "It was a differ-

ent generation," she says. "People worked harder physically back then, so they didn't feel the need for exercise. And women especially didn't do a lot of things outdoors."

Johnson began walking, dusting off a nonmotorized treadmill she had purchased long before her hypertension diagnosis. "I got it to lose some weight, but had used it sporadically," she admits. With the diagnosis, "I really had to use it now. My doctor reminded me that it was time to get serious about this."

So she did, walking about 20 minutes a day, usually five days a week. "When I exercise, I have

> **"Exercise sure beats taking pills for a lifetime."**

more energy and feel more on top of things," she says. "And I don't have that anxiety or heavy feeling that I often get with high blood pressure."

While her blood pressure fluctuates, it usually stays down around 130/70—good enough to remain medication-free. Johnson continues walking, and she does tai chi twice a week. The exercise may be a bitter pill to swallow, but at least it is not a real pill. And she is grateful she can do something about her BP.

Making Workouts Work

Only you know what can fire up your motivation and make your workouts work. But here are some final tips from the experts for getting—and staying—in shape:

Goal for it. Set both long-term health goals (like lowering your blood pressure or losing weight) and short-term exercise goals (like bicycling 10 miles or swimming half a mile). The latter will help you reach the former.

Stay real. If you're a big-boned person and come from a family with a history of obesity, it's unlikely that any amount of exercise will make you look as lean as television's sculpted *Baywatch* regulars. Remember: Even a 10 percent weight loss can significantly lower your blood pressure and reduce your risk for heart disease and other health problems.

Commit yourself. It's important to you and your family that you lower your blood pressure numbers and be as healthy as possible. In a real sense, your life depends on it. Make time for exercise. Pencil in your exercise sessions in your weekly planner, and think of them as compulsory, not optional, appointments.

Do it to music. Sign up for classes in swing dancing—or flamenco, folk, or African dance. All provide a terrific workout and a lot of fun. Or listen to music while you work out. Studies show that a musical beat gets you to work harder.

Gear to go. Make sure you have your exercise clothing and equipment handy and ready to use. That way you can take advantage of unexpected "down time" for a walk, bike ride, or other activity.

Tune in to your body. Ignore the old adage, "No pain, no gain." A strenuous workout may make your muscles "burn," but it should not—repeat, should not—cause pain. Stop exercising the moment you experience any kind of sharp pain. Ice, rest, and elevate the injured area, and call your doctor if the pain persists for more than a day or two.

Reward yourself. Whenever you've accomplished one of your short-term or long-term goals, celebrate! Treat yourself to a professional massage or manicure. Or buy yourself that CD you've wanted. But don't, of course, reward yourself with a fast-food milkshake or a plate of your favorite chocolate brownies!

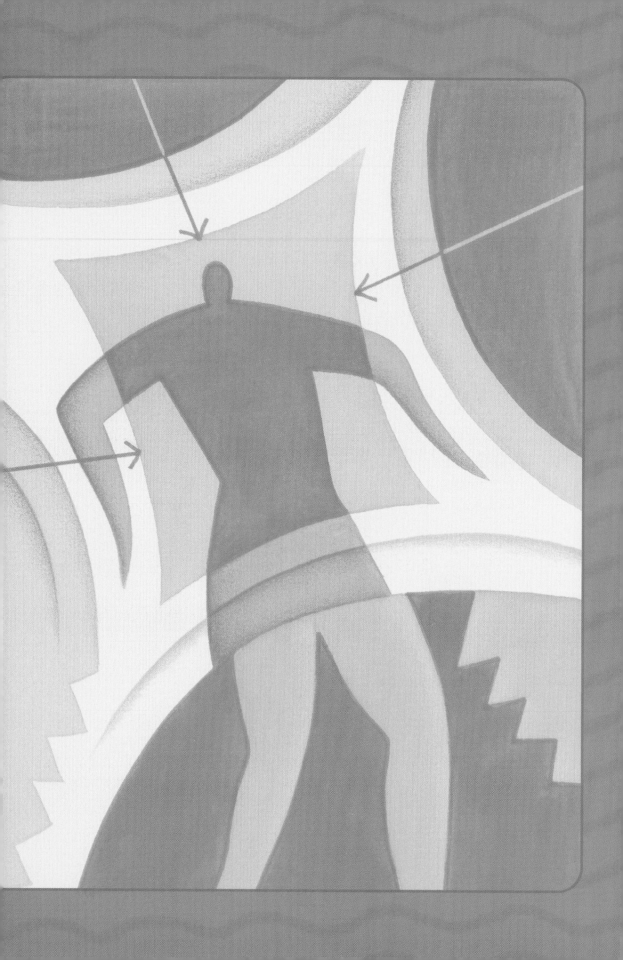

Don't Fret: Stifling Stress

Stress may or may not be a factor in high

blood pressure. Scientists just aren't sure. But

one thing is certain: Turning down the volume

on everyday stress and tension will help you

stick with the vital lifestyle changes needed to

lower your blood pressure.

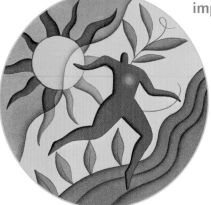

Just relax! Controlling stress can not only improve your overall health profile but also can provide the presence of mind to help you deflate your blood pressure numbers.

Busy, Busy, Busy

If you're like most of us, stress is no stranger. You may have a long, frustrating commute to and from work each day. You may have a workload that gets heavier with each passing year—and a boss who thinks it's not heavy enough.

Nor can you forget your work at home—all the laundry, cooking, shopping, cleaning, gardening, home repairing, bill-paying, and other chores that must be done and then redone, day after day, week after week. Then there are your kids, whose demanding schedules—packed daily with sports practices, dance classes, volunteer activities, homework assignments, and more—could rival that of any Fortune 500 CEO.

If your kids are grown, you may have other people—elderly parents, perhaps—who depend on you for financial and emotional support. Or you may have adult children, their lives in disarray, who have returned to live with you (along with their kids).

Now add to those relentless demands some of the big life stressors you've probably experienced over the years—things like a divorce, a disability, a move, a change in job, or even a chronic illness or death in the family. No wonder your blood pressure has steadily crept up, you tell yourself. Whose wouldn't?

Stress and HBP: Yes or No?

It's absolutely true that stress can elevate your blood pressure over the short run. Studies have shown that all sorts of activities, from arguing with a co-worker to cooking dinner, can cause a temporary spike in BP. Think about white-coat hypertension, detailed in Chapter 2: Just sitting in your doctor's office is enough to elevate your blood pressure into a higher realm. But can stress lead to sustained high blood pressure? Perhaps not. Contrary to popular thinking, scientists have been unable to prove any kind of consistent link between chronic stress and chronic hypertension.

> ➢ **Pressure Point:** If you experience stress
> regularly, the increases in blood pressure
> it produces can, over a period of time,
> damage your heart, arteries, brain,
> kidneys, and eyes—just as persistent
> high blood pressure can.

Still, if you have (or want to prevent) high blood pressure, it's important—some experts would say essential—to learn how to manage stress. The calmer and happier you feel, the more likely you are to make lifestyle changes, like eating well and exercising more, that can help you dramatically lower your blood pressure for good.

Think about it: When you're under a lot of stress, are you more or less likely to gorge on a candy bar from the vending machine or dip into a bag of some salty, high-fat snack food? And when you're loaded with worries or rushing around to meetings, your child's music lessons, or other must-do commitments, what are your chances of taking the time to exercise every day? Close to zero?

All of us, but especially those suffering from high blood pressure, need to s…l…o…w…d…o…w…n and de-pressurize our lives. In this chapter, you'll learn not only about personality traits that perhaps make you more susceptible to stress but also how stress burnout has more to do with how you process stress than with the outside stressors themselves.

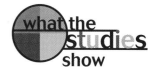

what the studies show

▶ *Lowering your cholesterol may give you better control over your blood pressure during times of stress. That's what researchers at the University of Rochester discovered. High cholesterol appears to make it more difficult for blood vessels to stay relaxed. And the tighter, or more constricted, your blood vessels become, the higher your blood pressure is likely to rise.*

Change Is Tough

Stress is the result of change—any change, good or bad. Finally getting a long-sought job promotion, for example, might be a good change in your life, but one that might also produce stress. Anything that takes you out of your ordinary routine and causes a state of emotional or physical tension is called stress.

An Emotional Throwback?

Could high blood pressure be the result of repressed emotions from childhood? That's the controversial theory of Samuel Mann, M.D., an internist at New York Presbyterian Hospital-Cornell Medical School. Mann believes that stifled emotional trauma from earlier life events may explain as many as a third of the adult cases of primary high blood pressure (the most common type of HBP—the one with no known causes).

Outing your memories. Many people with repressed emotions are highly resilient and appear emotionally strong on the surface, Mann says. But locked-away memories need to be expressed, and all too often, he says, they surface in toxic ways—such as by causing blood pressure to surge out of control. Mann recommends psychotherapy to many of his hypertensive patients and claims that such therapy often helps bring down their blood pressure.

Don't rush off to a psychoanalyst's couch quite yet, however. So far, Mann's evidence is only anecdotal, which is why many high blood pressure experts remain unconvinced by his very controversial theory. Rigorous studies would first need to be conducted to determine with any scientific certainty that deeply buried emotions can lead to high blood pressure.

Most of us, however, think only of gut-wrenching, teeth-gnashing stress. The word itself conjures up instant images of life's daily hassles—lost keys, traffic jams, work deadlines, endless meetings, money worries, and the like. Some of these negative stressors are external, or ones over which we have little control. You can't control, for example, if your child gets sick or if an airline decides to delay your flight. But many stressors are internal, or self-generated. You can control how you react when your boss criticizes your work or when the plumbing in your house suddenly breaks down. (You'll find out more about how to control your reactions to stress later in this chapter.)

When Stress Gets Physical

Your body is basically blind to the type of stress you are experiencing: It can't tell the difference between good and bad stressors. Both are perceived as a threat, and both trigger the same physiological response.

It's automatic. When you see or sense some kind of risk or danger, your brain immediately (and automatically) releases the "stress hormones" epinephrine and norepinephrine (also known as adrenaline and noradrenaline) as well as cortisol. These chemicals speed up your heartbeat—about two to three times its normal pace—and narrow your arteries, which, of course, raises your blood pressure. Blood (and oxygen) is rerouted from the skin and surface areas of the body to major muscles in your arms and legs, readying them for action. Your breathing also accelerates, your eyes dilate (to help you see better), and you may begin to sweat (to cool your body).

All these physical reactions are preparing your body to either fight the perceived threat or scurry away, which is why they are known collectively as the "fight-or-flight response." Because of this immediate and totally involuntary response, you can run faster, hit harder, jump higher, and see and hear better than under normal circumstances. You can also think faster. You become supercharged.

From tigers to traffic jams. For our prehistoric ancestors, the fight-or-flight response was essential. It increased the odds of surviving encounters with saber-tooth tigers and other life-threatening dangers. But once the hazard was dealt with—by either escaping it or conquering it—our cave-dwelling forebears immediately relaxed and went about their daily business. For them, stress was a short-lived phenomenon, the way nature intended it to be.

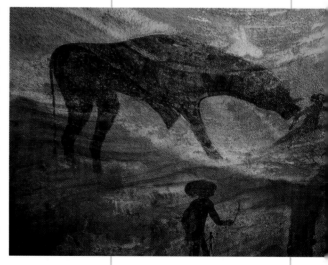

One, Two, Three—You're Stressed!

The Swiss-born endocrinologist and pioneer stress researcher Hans Selye (1907-1982) identified three distinct phases that people go through in response to stressful events.

Stage 1: The Alarm Phase

Your body recognizes the stress. It automatically triggers the fight-or-flight response, with all its physical symptoms (including increased heart rate and blood pressure, rapid breathing, and sweating). You experience an increase in energy. The pressure of the stress may cause you to feel excited or fearful.

Stage 2: The Resistance Phase

As the stress continues, your energy becomes depleted and you begin to feel overwhelming fatigue. Your body tries to repair damage caused during the alarm phase, but is unable to because of the persisting physiological demands of the stress. You become irritable and overreact to minor annoyances. You may also begin to feel anxious and have trouble sleeping. Other people notice these changes in you.

Stage 3: The Exhaustion Phase

If the stressful situation is not resolved, you eventually will become exhausted, or almost completely devoid of energy. Your body begins to succumb to both physical and mental stress-related illnesses, from headaches and heartburn to memory loss and depression. At this stage, stress can cause serious damage to your health. To avoid total burnout, you need to extract yourself from the stress or get help so that you can have some relief from it.

> **Pressure Point:** Studies have shown that as many as three out of four doctor visits are stress-related.

The saber-tooth tigers of modern life—family conflicts, rush-hour traffic jams, financial woes, and the like—rarely pose a danger to our physical survival. But they still elicit the fight-or-flight response. In most cases, however, it is impossible—and inappropriate—for us to either fight or flee. We can't punch out the department store salesperson who is rude to us, nor can we simply abandon a car on a congested freeway in the middle of rush hour (no matter how much temporary satisfaction such actions might bring!). Instead, we are taught from childhood to stay in control during such situations—in other words, to repress our natural fight-or-flight instincts.

Modern-day stress also tends to be continuous. The tigers (bills, chores, car problems—you name it) keep charging after us, day in and day out. When stressful situations go on for too long without any relief, both our physical and emotional health can suffer. We may develop headaches, backaches, stomach "problems," insomnia, fatigue, frequent colds, and more. We may also become irritable, discouraged, depressed, or even withdrawn.

Top 10 Causes of Stress

After conducting more than 5,000 interviews, researchers at the University of Washington School of Medicine identified the following top 10 stressors linked to illness or injury:

- Death of a spouse
- Divorce
- Marital separation
- Jail term
- Death of a close family member
- Personal injury or illness
- Marriage
- Involuntary job loss
- Marital reconciliation
- Retirement

According to Georgia Witkin, Ph.D., director of the stress program at Mount Sinai Medical Center in New York City, chronic stress can also contribute to what she calls the Four D's: disorganization, decision-making difficulties, depression, and dependency fantasies (wishing to be rescued by someone who makes everything all better).

Physical Symptoms of Stress

Short Term	Long Term
Rapid heartbeat	Headaches
Increase in blood pressure	Muscle aches
Rapid breathing	Heartburn
Excess sweating	Changes in appetite
Cold hands and feet	Frequent fatigue
Tense muscles	Reduced sex drive
Feelings of nausea or "butterflies in stomach"	Frequent colds and other illnesses
Diarrhea or urge to urinate	Insomnia
Dry mouth	
Dilation of eyes	

Emotional Symptoms of Stress

- Anger
- Anxiety
- Depression
- Fear
- Feeling abandoned
- Feeling isolated
- Grief
- Guilt
- Irritability

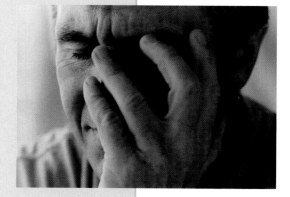

De-stress, don't distress. You can't, of course, eliminate all the stress in your life. Nor would you want to. Without some stress, many of us would have little incentive to do a good job at work, improve our personal relationships, contribute to our communities, and otherwise enrich and better our lives. But, whenever possible, you should try to reduce the number and/or the intensity of the stressors in your life.

And what if that's not possible? What do you do when faced with unavoidable stress, such as job loss or a storm-damaged roof? You try to change the way you respond to it. Such action is not always easy, but it is possible. Keep reading.

Are You Born to Be Stressed?

Scientists have been trying to determine for decades if people with certain personality types are more likely to develop high blood pressure. Some studies have found, for example, that people with hypertension tend to be more anxious and depressed than those with normal blood pressure. Other studies have looked at "type A" personalities—people who are aggressive, hostile, cynical, and ambitious—and found a similar link with high blood pressure. Still other studies have found that such characteristics as submissiveness, restrained aggression, and repressed inner tension are associated with HBP.

None of these studies has been conclusive, however, partly because methods used to categorize personalities vary. Some of the studies, for example, used standardized personality tests, but others didn't; some measured expressed anger, while others measured repressed anger; and so on. "White coat hypertension"—the tendency of many people's blood pressure to register "high" when in the doctor's office but not elsewhere—also may have skewed the studies' results.

Scientists are now coming to believe that the relationship between personality and high blood pressure may be more complex than previously understood. A recent study by researchers at State University of New York, Stony Brook, for example, measured a range of personality traits in 283 men, including anger, anger expression, anxiety, hopelessness, and submissiveness. To protect against white coat hypertension, the participants' blood pressure was monitored in several ways, including using a portable sphygmomanometer for 24 hours.

The study found that men with mild hypertension were no more likely to have particular personality characteristics than those with normal blood pressure. If personality does play a role in the development of high blood pressure, the study's authors speculated, it may be only to enhance or reduce the effects of a genetic predisposition to the condition.

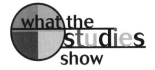
what the studies show

▶ *According to a study in the journal* Hypertension, *men with high levels of hopelessness—defined as a sense of futility and negative expectations about the future—were three times more likely to develop hypertension than those with low levels.*

The Big Chill: Anti-Stressing Strategies

Stress experts have countless strategies for preventing and reducing stress, from taking stock of your stress to taking deep breaths. Some of the most effective ones are described on the following pages. Which approaches will work for you? It all depends on your personality, your interests, and how willing you are to try something new.

Add Up Your Bothers

Identifying the symptoms of stress is the first step toward taking care of the problem. For many of us, however, stress has become such an ingrained part of our everyday world that we remain unaware of how perniciously it has invaded—and affected—our lives.

Running Hot

Some people are "hot reactors": In response to stress, they experience an extreme increase in blood pressure and heart rate. Dr. Robert Eliot, an American cardiologist and stress researcher, was the first to identify this group of people. He also was the first to suggest that hot reactors had a greater-than-average chance of developing high blood pressure later in life.

Several studies have supported Eliot's theory. In a recent study conducted at the University of North Carolina at Chapel Hill, for example, researchers found that how young adults respond to stress can help predict whether or not they'll have high blood pressure 10 years later. More than 100 male college students, aged 18 to 22, were recruited for the study. The students whose blood pressure and pulse increased the most during two stress tests (one mental, one physical) and who had at least one parent with high blood pressure were seven times more likely to develop high blood pressure a decade later than their peers who had neither of these risk factors.

Has stress become a problem in your life? Ask yourself these questions:

> Do you feel tense, anxious, panicky, or worried?

> Do you feel there is not enough time in the day?

> Do you have a hard time saying "no" without feeling guilty?

> Are you often impatient or irritable?

> Have you been forgetful or had difficulty concentrating?

> Are you smoking or drinking more than usual?

> Do you feel depressed or lack energy or interest in life?

> Do you find it difficult to make decisions?

> Are you always in a hurry?

> Do you seem to suffer from a lot of minor illnesses, such as colds, headaches, back pain, and stomach problems?

> Are you sleepy or tired during the day?

> Do you become impatient with delays or interruptions?

All of us experience these symptoms from time to time, but if any of the above statements describe how you feel most of the time, your stress level is probably too high.

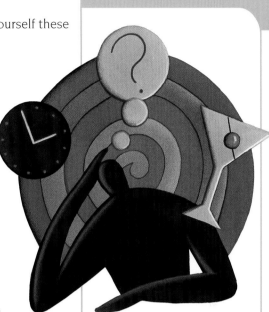

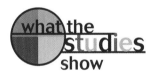

what the studies show

▶ *If you're anxious or depressed, your chances of developing high blood pressure over the next 10 years are double what it would be otherwise—or triple, if you're African American.*

Learn Optimism

In many cases, stress is a case of perception versus reality. It's how you perceive a particular situation—not necessarily the situation itself—that determines whether or not you'll become stressed out over it. Some people are natural optimists. They tend to look on the bright side of things, even when faced with difficult challenges and setbacks. Other people are pessimists. They tend to let stress get the best of them and react in a variety of destructive ways, from getting angry and physically or verbally abusive to becoming withdrawn and "giving up."

> **Pressure Point:** People who are pessimists tend to have higher blood pressure, according to a study conducted at the University of Michigan. A dreary attitude can also shorten your life. Researchers at the Mayo Clinic found that pessimists do indeed die younger than optimists.

The Write Way to Reduce Stress

Maintaining a stress diary is an effective way of finding out what causes you stress. In a special notebook or journal, record the following information at regular intervals—say, every three hours— over a period of several weeks.

- The date and time.

- The amount of stress that you are feeling at that particular time. (You can use a scale of 1 to 10, if you wish.)

- How happy or content you feel. (Again, use a scale of 1 to 10.)

Be sure to also record stressful events. Write down:

- The date and time of the event.

- What happened to cause the stress.

- The amount of stress that you felt.

- How you handled the event. Note whether you dealt with the cause of the stress or only with its symptoms.

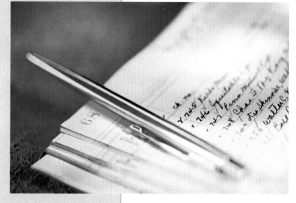

- Reflect on whether you handled the stress as effectively as possible. What else could you have done?

After a few weeks, you should have a clearer idea of what triggers your stress. Use that information to plan better strategies for de-stressing your life.

Are you a pessimist? Do you engage in a lot of negative "self-talk" that adds stress to your life (and raises your blood pressure)? You probably already know the answer to that question. But if you're unsure, think about a situation that frequently stresses you out—a rush-hour traffic jam, perhaps, or making a presentation at work. Try to recall your automatic thoughts at such moments. Do those thoughts fall into a predictable, negative pattern? Do they tend to exaggerate or distort the situation (rather than evaluate it realistically)? Also, do you find yourself blaming or deriding yourself for being caught in the stressful situation? If you answered "yes" to these questions, then chances are you are a pessimist.

Instant optimism. Pessimists can (and do!) learn how to replace negative, self-defeating, and irrational thoughts with positive, affirming ones. As a result, they can make great strides in minimizing stress's negative impact on their emotional and physical health. One technique recommended by experts at Harvard University's Mind Body Medical Institute involves four quick-and-simple steps: Stop. Breathe. Release. Reflect. With practice, these steps can help you redirect your thoughts—and behaviors—toward more positive outcomes.

Step 1: When you find yourself in a stressful situation, stop! Don't let your negative thoughts take control. Instead, immediately go to Step 2.

Step 2: Take several slow, deep breaths.

Step 3: As you breathe, relax your muscles and release tension.

Step 4: Now take a few moments to reflect on your negative thoughts. Are those thoughts contributing to the stress? Are they logical? Are they true? Where did you learn them? As you contemplate your answers, new and more positive thoughts should emerge.

Exorcise Tension with Exercise

Getting physical is one of the best and quickest ways to get rid of the epinephrine and other stress hormones that are pumped into your body during the fight-or-flight response. If you don't burn off those take-no-prisoner hormones, they can perpetuate

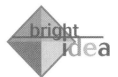

▶ *When you're feeling negative, try refocusing your thoughts on the positive. Jot down 5 to 10 things that make you happy, such as your marriage, your children, a friendship, a hobby, or a special place you like to visit. Reflect on them. Just thinking about things you enjoy can make you feel more content and less stressed.*

your tension—and elevate your blood pressure—for hours. Any kind of exercise will do—walking, running, swimming, even a strenuous weight-lifting workout. But avoid competitive sports, like tennis and racquetball, unless you find them fun and relaxing.

Regular aerobic exercise is also an effective long-term stress manager. It increases alpha activity in the brain, which is associated with tranquil moods. It raises the flow of endorphins, natural pain-relieving hormones that ease tension and boost mood. It relaxes tense muscles and helps induce deep, restorative sleep. Also, studies have shown that people who exercise before tackling stressful situations experience a smaller rise in blood pressure. For tips on how to build exercise into your lifestyle, see Chapter 4.

Perchance to dream. Even without a biochemical explanation, however, there are ample reasons why exercise has a beneficial effect on stress. When you exercise, you distance yourself from everyday pressures and are able to let your mind roam free; you feel more in control of your body and destiny. If you exercise outdoors, you have an opportunity to appreciate some of the natural beauty around you. All of this helps to control and counteract stress.

Carbs That Calm

Do you reach for the sweets when you're under stress? That may be because your body is craving the tranquilizing effects of

TV and Stress: Bad Reception

Watching TV may put you into a trancelike state, but does it reduce your stress? Not really, says Rutgers University psychologist Robert Kubey. His studies show that although sitting in front of the tube may increase alpha activity in the brain and other signs of calmness, the relaxed state quickly disappears as soon as the television is turned off. At that juncture, viewers usually feel sluggish, guilty, lonely, and generally dissatisfied—anything but calm and content, Kubey reports.

TV can be relaxing if you watch purposively, not mindlessly. Turn on the set only when you have a particular show you want to watch. Then, once that show is over, turn off the tube!

The Green Pharmacy

Calming kava. This popular herb relaxes skeletal muscles without depressing the central nervous system, leaving you calm yet alert. In studies it has been shown to work almost as well at quelling anxiety as tranquilizers and anxiety-reducing medications. Take no more than 250 mg a day, and don't take them for more than three months. Warning: Don't consume kava if you plan to drive.

Good ginseng. Panax ginseng is believed to reduce the harmful effects of stress, possibly by balancing the release of stress hormones. It may also enhance the production of endorphins, the body's feel-good hormones. The active ingredient is a compound called ginsenoside, which is extracted from the plant's root. Look for a brand standardized to contain at least 7 percent ginsenosides, and take 100 to 250 mg once or twice a day.

carbohydrates, say researchers at the Massachusetts Institute of Technology (MIT). Carbs trigger the release of the amino acid tryptophan into the brain, where it's converted into a soothing chemical called serotonin.

Sugar calms quickest, in about five minutes. Starches (including fruits, veggies, and bread) take about half an hour. If you decide on the quick fix, don't overdo it. Just a handful of jelly beans can induce tranquility. Also, don't reach for sweet rolls, cakes, ice cream, or other fat-ladened sweets; the fat can slow down the relaxation process by an hour or more. (It can also hinder your efforts to keep your weight—and thus your blood pressure—down.)

Because liquids get absorbed into the body faster than solids, the MIT researchers recommend drinking your carbs. Have a cup of instant cocoa (made with water or nonfat milk), or add a couple of tablespoons of sugar (the real stuff, not artificial substitutes or sweeteners) to a cup of decaffeinated coffee or herb tea.

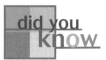

▶ *Listening to classical music can speed up the recovery from temporary jumps in high blood pressure brought on by stress. In one study, it took an average of 3.7 minutes for the participants' blood pressure to drop down to normal after performing a stressful task. But when they listened to the soothing classical tunes of Bach, Beethoven, Brahms, and the like, their blood pressure dropped almost one-quarter faster, or in an average of 2.9 minutes.*

Try a Musical Sedative

For more than 2,000 years, many people have subscribed to the theory that music can soothe the savage and stressful soul. The ancient Greek philosophers, for example, recommended that people either sing or play an instrument to rid themselves of their worries. And in the Bible, King Saul, Israel's first ruler, turned to harp music to lift his spirits.

> ▶**Pressure Point:** Modern science supports the age-old belief in music's ability to calm and comfort. Studies have shown that listening to music can reduce blood pressure and heart rate; it can also relax tired, tense muscles.

Go slow. Slow, quiet, instrumental music appears to be the best for soothing the stressed-out soul. The style of the music—rock, classical, folk, New Age, jazz, or other—doesn't matter, as long as you find it pleasing and calming. Be sure to focus fully on the sedative sounds; background music will do little for your nerves (or your blood pressure). Some music therapists recommend that you ease yourself into a more tranquil state by listening first to music that matches your initial, high-stressed mood (hard rock?), then switching to something slightly less agitated (an overture to a rousing Broadway musical?), before settling on a totally peaceful, calming composition, such as a slow movement from a Mozart or even a Chopin piano concerto.

The Sleep Solution

Here's a no-brainer: Getting a good night's sleep helps reduce stress. If you're chronically sleep-deprived—and, amazingly, two-thirds of Americans are—you'll be so tired during the day that you'll find it difficult to cope well with stressful situations.

Studies have also shown that being overtired can increase your blood pressure, especially when coupled with stress. One intriguing study of Long Island Railroad commuters, for example, found that people who had long commutes (more than 75 minutes) tended to have more daytime sleepiness and higher blood pressure than people with short commutes (less than 45 minutes).

> **Pressure Point:** Since 1910, the average number of hours people in developed countries sleep each night has dropped from 9 to 7.5.

Start thinking of a good night's sleep as a necessity, not a luxury. How much sleep do you need? That depends. It's not true that everyone needs eight hours of sleep. Some need more, some need less. Exactly how much you need is determined by your genes. You can shave off a little of your sleep requirement

A Sleep Clinic: The A to Zzzs of Better Sleep

- Avoid coffee and other caffeinated beverages for at least six hours before going to bed.

- Avoid alcohol for at least two hours before going to bed. Alcohol can make you feel more relaxed, but it can interfere with the quality of your sleep and cause frequent awakenings.

- Keep regular sleep hours—even on weekends. That means getting up at around the same time each morning, no matter how late you stayed up the night before.

- Nap judiciously. An occasional restorative nap can be a good thing. But don't nap if you have trouble sleeping at night.

- Do aerobic exercises regularly, preferably in the late afternoon or early evening (but not too close to bedtime).

- Quit smoking. People who smoke have greater difficulty both falling and staying asleep.

- Don't toss and turn. If you don't fall asleep within 30 minutes, get up and go to another room. Read or sit quietly until you feel sleepy, then return to bed.

- Don't rely on sleeping pills. Such medications should be used for short bouts of insomnia, not for chronic sleep problems.

and be none the worse for it, but if you start cutting back on your sleep by an hour or more, you'll start to feel it. Almost immediately. You'll become cranky and irritable, your mental and physical skills will diminish, and even a little bit of stress will suddenly seem like a big deal.

Sleep Apnea: It's More Than a Snore

High blood pressure and sleep apnea—a serious, potentially life-threatening condition in which breathing is repeatedly interrupted during sleep—are strongly linked, studies have shown. In fact, people with moderate to severe sleep apnea are almost seven times more likely to have high blood pressure than those without apnea, according to research from the Pennsylvania State University College of Medicine in Hershey.

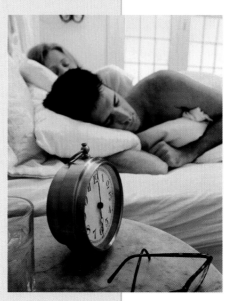

Many people are unaware they have sleep apnea until told by their bed partners or family members that they are snoring heavily and struggling for breath throughout the night. Debilitating daytime sleepiness is also a sign of the condition. If you suspect you have sleep apnea, be sure to discuss it with your doctor. Sleep apnea can be treated, often with the use of a continuous positive airway pressure device, which delivers a steady stream of air into the nasal passages through a mask that is worn during sleep.

Fascinating footnote: The study also found a link between simple snoring and high blood pressure. People who don't have apnea but who snore are one-and-a-half times more likely to have HBP than those who don't snore.

Muscling In on Stress

To neutralize the fight-or-flight stress response, try progressive muscle relaxation. This technique, which has been found to reduce high blood pressure as well as stress and anxiety, is based on the simple idea of tensing and then releasing groups of muscles one at a time. Here's how to do it.

> Lie in a comfortable position on a thick carpet or exercise mat. (You can also sit, if you wish.) Close your eyes.

> Breathe in deeply. As you do so, tense your entire body and hold the tension for a few seconds. Then exhale and release the tension. Notice how different your body feels.

> Starting with your feet, tense and then release one muscle group at a time. Move progressively up your body: After your feet, tense and release your calves, then your thighs, buttocks, stomach, and so on. Be sure to include your facial muscles.

> When you've finished, lie quietly for a moment. Your whole body should feel warm (from the increase in blood flow to the muscles) and relaxed.

Practice this technique daily or whenever you find yourself in a stressful situation.

A Tranquilizer without Side Effects

Meditation, performed for thousands of years as part of many religious practices, can lower stress-hormone levels, heart rate, and blood pressure, modern scientists have discovered. It can also slow down brain waves, causing them to enter the calming alpha state or sometimes even the theta (or most relaxed wakeful) state. No wonder then that meditation has been described as "a tranquilizer without the side effects."

There are many different types of meditation. Two of the best known are transcendental meditation (TM), in which you focus your attention on silently repeating a mantra (a self-selected word or phrase), and mindfulness meditation, in which you quietly focus on your thoughts or emotions without judging or reacting to them.

Much of the research on meditation and blood pressure involve transcendental meditation. In one study, people with high blood pressure who practiced this technique not only lowered their blood pressure and pulse rate but also widened their arteries. No such benefits were seen in a control group of people with high blood pressure who engaged in relaxing leisure activities instead of meditation.

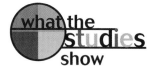

what the studies show

► *According to studies conducted in Norway, massage increases blood levels of endorphins, your body's own mood-elevating, stress-relieving compounds. Whether the massage was given by a friend or yourself, the results were equally beneficial.*

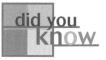

did you know

► *Levels of the stress hormone cortisol rise more steeply on Monday morning than on other workday mornings, suggesting that just the anticipation of work triggers job-related stress.*

Another study of 111 middle-aged and elderly African-American men and women showed that transcendental meditation lowered blood pressure more significantly than progressive muscle relaxation or an education program encouraging people to adopt more healthful lifestyle habits. After three months, the meditation practitioners experienced an average drop in systolic pressure of 10.7 mm Hg and in diastolic pressure of 6.5 mm Hg—about twice the drop seen in the study participants who practiced progressive muscle relaxation. For those who underwent the education program to change their lifestyle, the news wasn't good at all: They actually experienced an increase in blood pressure.

Meditation by the Numbers: Five Easy Pieces

You can get started by doing the following basic transcendental meditation exercise for 15 to 20 minutes, once or twice a day.

1 Sit comfortably, preferably in a quiet place.

2 Close your eyes. Breathe naturally for about a minute as you allow your mind and body to calm.

3 Take slow, deep breaths. As you exhale, silently repeat a word or phrase—any one you choose. Some people select a neutral word, such as "one" or "om." Others prefer an inspirational word, such as "peace" or "love." Still others opt for a religious phrase or prayer, such as "The Lord is my shepherd."

4 When thoughts intrude (and they will!), avoid any attempt to control them. Just make note of them and then gently try to return to your mantra. You may find this step difficult at first, but over time it will become easier to let go of your thoughts and enter a state of deep relaxation.

5 When you are done, take a minute to return to awareness. Rise and reenter the world slowly.

After several weeks of practice, you'll likely discover that in addition to being more relaxed after meditating, you'll also be calmer at other times of the day.

Take a Deep Breath

When we're feeling stressed, we tend to take short, shallow, irregular breaths that fill only our upper chests with oxygen. We may even, without realizing it, hold our breath. This kind of breathing decreases the amount of oxygen circulating in our blood. The heart then reacts by pumping more blood (to get more oxygen into the body), which then, of course, raises blood pressure.

You can cope better with stress and perhaps lower your blood pressure by breathing more deeply. Deep, or diaphragmatic, breathing also reduces muscle tension and promotes relaxed alertness.

Practice the following technique once a day and whenever you find yourself under particular stress.

> Make yourself comfortable. Either sit in a straight chair or lie on your back with your feet slightly apart.

> Close your eyes. Place your hand on your stomach just below the navel. This will help you make sure that you are breathing from your abdomen, not from your upper chest.

> Breathe in slowly through your nose. (If your nose is congested, breathe in through your mouth, with lips slightly parted.) Count slowly as you breathe: Inhale (one, two, three, four). Imagine energy and calmness entering your body with the breath. You should feel the hand you placed on your stomach rise as you inhale.

> Hold the breath as you count to four again: Hold (one, two, three, four).

> Exhale slowly, again to the count of four: Exhale (one, two, three, four). Imagine tension leaving your body with the air. Your hand should fall as you exhale.

> Repeat the breathing for as long as 20 minutes, if you have the time. Gradually, as you become more relaxed, you may be able to increase the count up to eight for each breath.

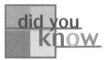

did you know

▶ *A bad marriage may be bad for your blood pressure. A study of more than 100 men and women found that people who reported being unhappy in their marriage were likely to have higher blood pressure three years later, while those people who expressed marital contentment were likely to see their blood pressure go down during that same period.*

Breathing Lessons

The FDA recently approved a new medical device, called a RespeRate, that coaches people with high blood pressure through a 15-minute deep-breathing session. Looking like a slightly enlarged portable compact disc player, the RespeRate includes a sensor, which is strapped around your waist, and headphones. The device uses the sensor to analyze your breathing patterns and then creates sound patterns to guide you to inhale and exhale at a slower pace.

Studies have shown that the RespeRate can lower systolic pressure by an average of 12 mm Hg and diastolic pressure by an average of 8 mm Hg after only six weeks of daily treatment. Don't hold your breath waiting to see the device at your local drugstore, however. Right now, the RespeRate is available only by doctor's prescription.

More Tension Tamers

Get a pet. Just being around animals can reduce anxiety and stress for many people. Evidence indicates that pets also help reduce blood pressure. In fact, one study showed that simply stroking a cat or dog can be enough to cause blood pressure to plummet—yours and your pet's.

Avoid caffeine. Coffee and other caffeinated beverages and products can raise blood pressure, especially when you're under stress. (More about caffeine and blood pressure in Chapter 6.)

Speak softly. Studies have shown that if your words spew forth loudly and rapidly, your blood pressure will rise, no matter what the topic. On the other hand, speaking softly and slowly—even about topics that anger you—will help keep your blood pressure on a low and even keel.

Stretch daily. Stretching is one of the all-time great tension relievers. (For descriptions of exercises you could start doing today, see Chapter 4.)

De-clutter your home. Having too much stuff can be a terrible source of stress. Throw out (or donate to charity) the stuff you don't use, and be more judicious about future purchases.

Share time with friends. According to polls, most of us prefer to be alone when we're under stress. You'd be wiser, however, to share your troubles with a good friend. Consider a study conducted on people undergoing heart catheterization, a difficult and stressful medical procedure. The study found that people who held the hand of a trusted friend during the procedure experienced a lower increase in blood pressure than those who underwent the procedure alone. Another study conducted at the University of Zurich, Switzerland, found that men who had their best friend with them when giving an unprepared speech or doing mental arithmetic in front of an audience had lower levels of stress hormones in their bodies than men who performed those tasks without a friend in attendance.

Laugh more. Humor can cut through tension like a hot knife through butter. It helps relax muscles, lower blood pressure (perhaps by getting more oxygen into your bloodstream), and may also lower the levels of stress hormones circulating in the body. So find something that makes you laugh—the comics in your morning paper, a movie starring your favorite comedian, a humor book, or the company of one or more fun-loving friends—and enjoy a good giggle or belly laugh. Do it today and every day, as often as you can.

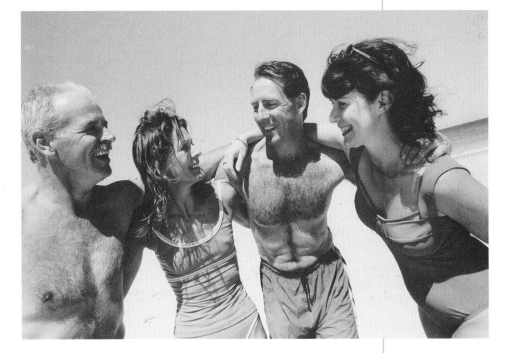

6 Taking Habits to Heart

For many people, the little pleasures of life

can be counted on one hand: a cup of coffee

with breakfast, a glass of wine or beer with

dinner, or a cigarette here and there. Taking

charge of your blood pressure will mean that

you can enjoy two out of three of those

habits—in moderation, of course.

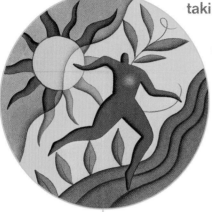

Taking charge of your high blood pressure means taking charge of your everyday habits—namely, drinking, smoking, and consuming caffeine.

Clearing the Smoke

On the face of it, the evidence for smoking causing high blood pressure might not seem convincing enough to get you to extinguish your butts. After all, the studies have shown that smoking raises blood pressure only temporarily, not permanently.

But don't flick your Bic quite yet. Step back and look at the bigger picture. Smoking (or any kind of tobacco use) may not be a direct cause of chronic high blood pressure, but it is definitely a major risk factor for cardiovascular disease—as is, of course, having high blood pressure. Combining the two creates an especially deadly duo. Statistics show that if you have high blood pressure and smoke, you are three to five times more likely to die of a heart attack and two times more likely to die of a stroke than if you didn't smoke.

➢**Pressure Point:** Health surveys show that 35 percent of hypertensive men and 33 percent of hypertensive women of all ages are smokers.

What Happens When You Inhale?

Your blood pressure rises every time you smoke. As soon as you take a puff, nicotine from the tobacco enters your bloodstream through the tiny blood vessels in your lungs. Within 10 seconds the nicotine shoots to your brain, which immediately signals your adrenal glands to release the hormone epinephrine (adrenaline). Just as with the fight-or-flight stress response, the epinephrine causes your blood vessels to narrow and your heart to pump harder (by as much as 25 beats per minute). This, of course, sends your blood pressure sky-high, at least for a time.

Can Smoking Lower Your HBP?

Some research suggests that smoking may lower blood pressure. One study found, for example, that women who are light smokers (smoking anywhere from one to nine cigarettes a day) actually tend to have lower blood pressure than women who are heavy smokers or who don't smoke at all.

There is an explanation: The women's blood pressure was lower probably because they weighed less. Nicotine suppresses appetite and speeds up metabolism, which means people tend to burn more calories throughout the day when they're using tobacco than when they're not. As a result, they carry around less body fat than if they didn't smoke. The more people weigh, the greater their chance of developing high blood pressure.

Pounds versus disease. But that doesn't mean you should take up smoking to control your blood pressure! The health risks of smoking are far greater than the risks of gaining a few pounds when you give it up—even if those extra pounds cause your blood pressure to creep up. Nor do you have to gain weight when you quit smoking. You can always take steps to eat sensibly and rev up your exercise sessions to keep the pounds off.

How high? Studies have shown that after smoking just two cigarettes, both systolic and diastolic blood pressures increase by an average of about 10 mm Hg—and they stay elevated for 15 to 30 minutes. So if you're a heavy smoker—your blood pressure could remain elevated most of your waking day.

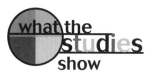

what the studies show

► *One study, conducted by researchers from Wake Forest University in Winston-Salem, North Carolina, found that atherosclerosis progressed 50 percent faster in smokers than nonsmokers. There was also bad news for nonsmokers who hung out with smokers for more than one hour per week: Their arteries hardened about 20 percent faster than people who restricted themselves to smoke-free environments.*

> **Pressure Point:** The nicotine from chewed tobacco takes three to five minutes to reach the brain and trigger the physiological responses that raise blood pressure.

Other negatives. Smoking aggravates your blood pressure in other ways as well. The chemicals in tobacco (and there are thousands) can scar the lining of your arteries, which can contribute to an artery-narrowing buildup of fatty plaque. Also, certain hormones triggered by tobacco can cause your body to retain above-normal levels of fluid. Both of these factors have the potential of raising your blood pressure over the long term.

Why You Should Stop (As If You Didn't Know)

There's no gentle way of saying this (nor should there be): Half of the people who smoke die from smoking-related diseases. They die, on average, 10 to 12 years earlier than their nonsmoking peers. In fact, smoking cigarettes is responsible for one of every five premature deaths in the United States, including:

> 20 percent of all deaths from cardiovascular disease

> 29 percent of all cancer deaths

> 87 percent of all lung cancer deaths

But if preventing your early death isn't enough of a reason to give up smoking once and for all, considering these additional incentives might do the trick:

> You'll have fewer wrinkles as you age.

> You'll have more energy.

> Your hair, clothes, house, and car will smell better. So will your breath.

> Your teeth and nails will lose that yellowish nicotine stain.

> Your favorite foods will smell and taste better.

As Time Goes By: What Happens When You Quit

Within hours of quitting your tobacco habit, your body will start healing itself. Here's some of what you can expect:

After 30 minutes: Your pulse rate slows down and your blood pressure drops.

After 12 hours: The level of carbon monoxide in your blood decreases, enabling the blood to carry more oxygen. You may notice you can do more physically demanding activities without becoming short of breath.

After 2 days: Nerve endings begin to recover and your sense of taste and smell begin to return.

After 1 week: Most physical withdrawal symptoms are gone (although psychological ones may remain).

After 2 weeks to 3 months: Your circulation improves. Your lung function improves by up to 30 percent.

Within 2 months: Blood flow returns to your hands and feet, keeping them warmer. Your skin appears healthier.

Within 3 months: The tiny, hairlike cells in the lungs called cilia, which your former smoking damaged, regrow. As a result, your lungs become more resistant to infection (because the cilia clean the lungs of organisms, irritants, and other debris). You may experience increased coughing for a few days, however, as the cilia rid your lungs of excess mucus.

Within 1 to 9 months: Fatigue and shortness of breath decrease, and you have more energy.

Within 1 year: Your risk for heart disease drops to half of what it was when you smoked.

Within 5 years: Your risk for lung cancer drops to half of what it was when you smoked.

Within 10 to 15 years: Your risk for lung cancer and heart disease drops to that of someone who has never smoked.

> Men only: You'll lower your risk of becoming impotent.

> If you're a woman, you'll lower your risk of developing osteoporosis (a condition in which bones gradually weaken and thin) or experiencing an early menopause.

> If you're pregnant, you'll increase your chances of having a healthy baby.

> The people (and pets!) you live with will be healthier.

Kicking the Habit

If you smoke, you've probably already tried to quit. Most people make several serious attempts at giving up smoking before they finally succeed. After all, nicotine is an addictive drug—for some people, as addictive as heroin or cocaine.

So it's no surprise that quitting is hard. Very hard. But each year, more than 3 million smokers do what many of them thought was impossible and give up cigarettes for good. You can do it, too! All it takes is the right attitude, knowledge, and planning.

Calling It Quits

There are many ways to quit smoking. Below are some of the most popular. For the greatest success, consider combining one of these methods with nicotine-replacement treatment (see p. 174) and stop-smoking counseling.

Cold turkey. With this method, you simply stop, suddenly and totally. For most people, this is the most successful way of kicking the nicotine habit.

Cutting down. Gradually reduce the amount of nicotine in your body by cutting down on the number of cigarettes you smoke each day—that is the essence of this approach. People usually eliminate 5 to 10 cigarettes a day until they can go "cold turkey" and quit altogether. Although some people have success with this method, studies have shown that most people lose their determination before reaching the quitting day.

Delay. This approach encourages you to put off the first cigarette of the day by one or two hours. Then each day you delay that first cigarette a little longer until you're not smoking any cigarettes. Delaying works for some people, but experts recommend you take no more than two weeks to be smoke-free.

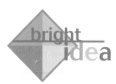

● *Smokers who survive a heart attack have the highest rate of success at quitting—they're extremely motivated! Of course, waiting until you have a close brush with death to kick your tobacco habit is not a great idea. You need to find motivation now. Make a list of your personal reasons for quitting. Carry the list with you so you can pull it out whenever you feel the urge to smoke.*

No matter which approach you choose, one thing is absolutely essential: You'll need a plan like the following one.

Step 1: Get ready

Start by picking a specific quit date. Make sure it's not so far away that you soon forget about it, or so close that you won't have time to properly prepare. Some people choose a day when they're on vacation and away from their regular routine (easier to break old smoking habits). Others prefer to quit on a typical and more structured day (easier to keep busy and distracted from smoking). Whichever type of day you choose, be sure it's one that is relatively free of stress. Circle it on your calendar.

Replay your strategy. Next, review your past attempts at quitting. What worked and what didn't? Think in particular about the situations that make you want a cigarette. Perhaps you always light up after a meal or as soon as you get in your car. Start preparing for what you'll do instead of smoking in

Weathering Withdrawal

By stopping smoking, you're cutting off your body's supply of the addictive drug nicotine. As a result, you'll experience strong physical cravings and withdrawal symptoms. Although unpleasant, these symptoms are actually good news. They mean your body is clearing itself not only of nicotine but also of tobacco's other toxins. Below you'll find the major symptoms—and what you can do to get relief from them.

Symptom	How Long	What You Can Do
Dry mouth/sore throat	A few days	Sip cold water or fruit juice; chew gum.
Coughing	A few days	Sip warm herbal tea; suck on cough drops or hard candy.
Constipation	1 to 2 weeks	Add fiber to your diet (fruits, vegetables, and whole grains); drink plenty of water.
Headache	1 to 2 weeks	Take a warm bath or shower; try meditation or other tension-relieving techniques; drink plenty of water.
Hunger	1 to 4 weeks	Eat regular meals; snack on low-fat, low-calorie foods; drink plenty of water.
Tenseness / irritability	2 to 4 weeks	Exercise regularly; practice meditation and other tension-relieving techniques; take a warm bath or shower.
Fatigue	2 to 4 weeks	Take naps when needed; avoid doing too much and overstressing yourself.
Difficulty sleeping	2 to 4 weeks	Avoid caffeine after 6:00 P.M.; practice stress-reducing techniques (see chapter 5); exercise regularly (but not too close to bedtime).

Nicotine without Smoke: How Aids Can Help

Nicotine-replacement products can greatly increase your odds of quitting smoking. They send a controlled amount of nicotine to your brain, which is gradually reduced until you are weaned from the drug altogether. Research has shown that people are most successful at quitting smoking when they combine the use of nicotine-replacement products with counseling that focuses on changing behavior. Nicotine-replacement products come in the following forms:

Nicotine patches, which can be purchased without a prescription, deliver a measured dose of nicotine through the skin. They are available in several dosages and are generally used for 6 to 12 weeks.

Cautions: The most common side effects are mild skin irritation (if so, try different brands) and insomnia (if so, switch to a lower dose patch or take off the patch at night).

Nicotine gum delivers its nicotine through the mucous membranes of the mouth within about 20 minutes. It is available in two strengths and can be bought without a prescription. One of the advantages of nicotine gum is that you control the dose; one of its disadvantages is that it's easy to become dependent on it and to continue using it past the recommended six-month limit.

Cautions: Side effects can include soreness in the mouth (usually from chewing the gum the wrong way), hiccups, and upset stomach.

Nicotine nasal sprays are available only by prescription. They deliver nicotine into the bloodstream through the nasal mucous membranes within 5 to 10 minutes, which makes them very useful in overcoming immediate nicotine cravings.

Cautions: The most common side effects include nose and throat irritation, watery eyes, sneezing, and coughing. Sprays should not be used for more than six months, and their use should be tapered at the end of three months. They are often not recommended for people with asthma, allergies, nasal polyps, or sinus problems.

Nicotine inhalers require a prescription. They consist of a plastic rod with a nicotine plug. When you puff on the inhaler, the plug produces a nicotine vapor that is absorbed into the bloodstream within about 20 minutes, primarily through the mouth.

Cautions: Common side effects include coughing and mouth and throat irritation.

those situations. You could plan to go for a short walk after meals, for example, or to chew gum (from packets conveniently stashed in your car's glove compartment) when driving.

Work also on visualizing what it will be like to stop smoking. Imagine how much better you'll feel (more energized) and look (healthier and more attractive). Combining this visualization exercise with meditation or deep breathing (see page 162) can be especially effective in helping you quit.

Step 2: Rally support

Inform everyone you know—your family, your friends, your co-workers—that you have chosen a date to stop smoking. Tell them you'd like their support. Ask those who smoke not to do so when you're around. You may even find that one of those smokers will quit with you. Enlisting a quitting "buddy" can be a very effective motivator.

Make an appointment with your doctor to discuss different strategies for quitting, including nicotine and non-nicotine aids. You should also check with your health insurance plan to see what kind of stop-smoking strategies it supports and covers.

> **Pressure Point:** Research has shown that the more counseling you get, the better your chances of quitting.

Step 3: Create new routines

To help you make the psychological break from smoking, change as many of your daily routines as possible when you first quit. Take a different route to work, for example, or drink tea instead of coffee at your midmorning break. Getting out of your daily rut will help stop the urge to automatically light up a cigarette at certain moments in your day.

Start exercising. Studies have shown that people who exercise regularly are more successful at quitting smoking. Increasing physical activity will also help you counter any weight gain you might experience as a result of tossing away your tobacco. It will also improve your mood and help take off the edge of such withdrawal symptoms as irritability and headaches.

Reduce stress. If you were like most smokers, you probably used cigarettes to combat stress. Now you need to find other

did you know

▶ *With clinical trials beginning next winter, NicVAX—a nicotine vaccine—is four years away from readiness. But its potential is breathtaking: You get an injection; the drug stimulates antibodies to bind with the nicotine from your cigarette, preventing it from reaching your brain. The effects last for a year or two.*

ways of relieving tension. Exercise will help a lot, but you may also want to try meditation, deep breathing, or progressive muscle relaxation. (You'll find how-to details about all these techniques in Chapter 5.)

Practice positive self-talk. Congratulate yourself for making the effort to quit smoking. And try to stay focused on the positive, or what you're gaining from not smoking (check that list you made!), rather than on the negative, or the struggle you're having with nicotine withdrawal.

Quick Quit Tips

▪ Eat regular meals. Hunger can increase the urge to smoke.

▪ Take two deep breaths whenever you feel the need to smoke. Envision your lungs filling with fresh, clean air.

▪ If you feel that you are going to light up, tell yourself that you must wait at least 10 minutes. Often, the immediate urge to smoke will pass within that time frame.

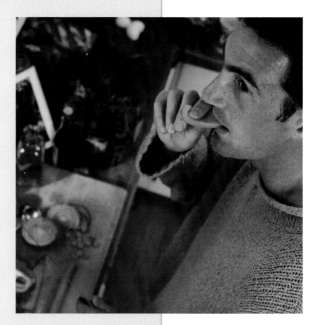

▪ Distract yourself when you get a nicotine craving. Do something else immediately—talk to a friend, go for a quick walk, or do some stretching exercises. Or go to a place (like the movies) where you're not allowed to smoke.

▪ Avoid "high-risk" places or situations—the ones that you connect with smoking.

▪ Reduce or avoid alcohol.

▪ Drink plenty of water and juices.

▪ Carry other things—gum, candy, carrot sticks, sunflower seeds, cinnamon sticks, toothpicks—to put in your mouth when you get the urge to smoke.

▪ Don't smoke—not even one puff!

No-Nicotine Medication

The prescription drug bupropion hydrochloride, sold under such brand names as Zyban and Wellbutrin, has been successfully used either alone or in combination with nicotine-replacement products to help people quit smoking. The medication increases the blood levels of dopamine, a natural chemical that not only improves mood but also helps battle nicotine cravings.

In one study, 49 percent of people who used Zyban were able to kick their smoking habit within one month compared to 36 percent of those who used the nicotine patch. But when people used both Zyban and the patch, 58 percent remained smoke-free for at least a month.

Hug yourself. Be kind to yourself. Plan something enjoyable to do every day. And don't forget to reward yourself at regular intervals for your spectacular effort at quitting. Treat yourself to a professional therapeutic massage, for example, or a new exercise outfit, or a low-fat yogurt "smoothie" at your favorite juice bar. You'll be able to afford such little extravagances now that you're saving money from not smoking!

Step 4: Hang in there!

Quitting is a one-day-at-a-time kind of effort. Be prepared for a possible relapse, especially during the first week when withdrawal symptoms tend to be strongest. If you do stumble and have a relapse, don't get discouraged. Take these steps instead:

> Don't be too hard on yourself. Having a slip-up and smoking one cigarette doesn't make you a smoker again.

> Get back on track immediately. Remind yourself why you quit and think about the effort you've already invested in quitting. Then reaffirm your commitment to giving up tobacco for good.

> Identify what caused you to break your resolve not to smoke again. Decide now what you'll do when the situation comes up again. For ideas and support, you may want to talk over your setback with a friend or professional.

> **Pressure Point:** When you're trying to quit, stay away from people who smoke. Three-quarters of quitters who relapse do so in the presence of smokers— usually after asking one of the smokers for a cigarette.

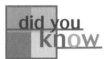

did you **know**

▶ *Nicotine can interfere with medications prescribed for high blood pressure. So always be honest with your doctor about your smoking (or tobacco-chewing) habits.*

Rethink Your Drinking

The media and the medical community have sent markedly mixed messages about alcohol. For years, we were told it was best not to drink. Lately, however, scientists have started reporting that wine and even other alcoholic beverages offer some protection against heart disease.

In the spring of 2001, for example, two respected studies suggested that consuming about seven alcoholic drinks per week might not only lower your risk for heart attack but might also raise your chance of surviving such an attack, should you have one. A lot of people could be heard saying, "I'll drink to that."

It may be a bit too hasty, however, to pop a celebratory cork. Although a growing number of studies seem to indicate that moderate (and that's the key word) drinking can protect your heart, none of these findings should be construed as a license to drink. That's especially true for people with high blood pressure.

> **Pressure Point:** Experts estimate that heavy alcohol use causes 5 to 11 percent of all cases of high blood pressure.

A Toast to Your Blood Pressure?

Large amounts of alcohol—wine, beer, vodka, whiskey, you name it—raise blood pressure. Studies have found that if you have three or more drinks a day, your systolic blood pressure is likely to rise by 3 to 4 mm Hg and your diastolic pressure by 1 to 2 mm Hg. If you swill down five or more drinks daily, your blood pressure may climb even higher—by 5 to 6 mm Hg for systolic and 2 to 4 mm Hg for diastolic.

Less is more. But having only one or two shots of tequila or glasses of Beaujolais per day doesn't appear to have any upward effect on blood pressure. In fact, studies have shown that people who indulge in one or two drinks a day have, on average, slightly lower blood pressure than nondrinkers. In addition, moderate levels of alcohol appear to elevate "good" HDL cholesterol—the kind that helps protect against heart disease.

The French Paradox: Beyond Beaujolais

For non-Francophiles, the so-called French paradox has seemed terribly unfair: How could people from France have lower rates of obesity and heart disease when their daily menus include butter, cream, foie gras, an endless array of pastry, cheese, and other high-fat gastronomical pleasures?

At first, baffled scientists believed the paradox could be explained by red wine, which contains an antioxidant called resveratrol (also found in purple grape juice) that may help protect the cardiovascular system from damage. Recently, however, scientists have found that alcohol itself, not resveratrol, raises levels of HDL, or "good," cholesterol, and thus reduces the risk of blood clotting, which can lead to heart attacks and strokes.

So wine may be only one factor in the French paradox. Perhaps a stronger explanation for the paradox may be found in the French diet. In France (and in other Mediterranean countries where the incidence of heart disease is low), people load up their plates with fresh fruits and vegetables and cook with monounsaturated fats, especially olive oil. They also drink less milk and serve smaller portions of meat at their meals. And—Americans take note!—they aren't as obsessed with high-fat, high-sodium snack foods.

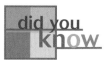

did you know

▶ *The mechanism by which excessive alcohol raises blood pressure is unknown, but scientists think that too much alcohol may release the hormone epinephrine, which constricts blood vessels.*

▶ *Genetics may determine whether or not alcohol triggers a rise in your blood pressure. Researchers have found that when genetically different strains of mice are fed the same amount of alcohol, some strains experience an increase in BP while others undergo a decrease.*

If you're a very heavy drinker, you'll be doing your blood vessels and heart (not to mention other important body organs, like your liver) a favor by cutting back on your alcohol consumption. One group of English researchers found, for example, that when men who tended to stay too long at the pub (those who consumed six to eight drinks per day) gave up ale and bitters completely, their blood pressure sank by 13 (systolic) and 5 mm Hg (diastolic) within four days. Once the men resumed their drinking, their blood pressure shot back up.

Another study had a group of men with high blood pressure cut back from four drinks a day to two. Their systolic blood pressure, which had ranged from 140 to 179 mm Hg, dropped an average of 3.6 points.

But what if you're a moderate drinker—a man who downs no more than a couple of beers or a woman who sips on no more than a single glass of wine each evening? Will cutting back on your alcohol lower your blood pressure? The studies so far suggest that the answer is no.

Watch your drinking. But there are other reasons to watch—and maybe reduce—your alcohol intake. Even light drinking has been linked to cirrhosis and cancer of the liver, several other cancers (of the breast, mouth, throat, and esophagus), hemorrhagic stroke, and osteoporosis. Alcohol can also have a profound effect on the brain, dulling memory, judgment, coordination, and reaction time. In addition, it can lead to depression, sexual dysfunction, and severe sleep disruptions. All of these are sobering reasons to reconsider your drinking habits.

What's in a Drink?

A standard drink is:

- **12 oz. of beer (regular or lite)**
- **3.5 oz. of wine**
- **1.5 oz. of 80-proof distilled spirits**
- **1 oz. of 100-proof distilled spirits**

Heavy drinking is defined as more than two drinks per day for men and more than one drink per day for women.

Deciding to Drink (or Not)

If you have high blood pressure and like to drink, you probably can continue do so—in moderation. In fact, it might even offer some protection against heart disease. But moderation is the key. That means no more than one (for women) or two (for men) drinks a day. (Small men and large women take note: This recommendation is based on body size, not gender.) If you drink anything more than that, your blood pressure is likely to increase—and with it your risk for heart disease. Of course, anyone with a past history of alcoholism shouldn't drink at all.

> **CAUTION**
>
> If you're a heavy drinker who wants to cut back, do so gradually over a period of a week or two. A sudden decrease in alcoholic consumption can trigger a big release of epinephrine, which can lead to a severe—and potentially dangerous—surge in blood pressure that could last for several days.

By the way, don't think you can save up some of those daily drinks and then "spend" them all at once at a party or bar on Saturday night. Binge drinking offers no health benefits—only an increased chance of dying prematurely, perhaps from a heart attack. When you do a lot of drinking at once (more than three drinks per occasion for women or more than four for men), you can develop an irregular heartbeat and spike your blood pressure, which might trigger a heart attack.

And what if you're a happy teetotaler? Stay that way! There are more effective—and, frankly, less risky—ways than drinking to lower your risk for heart disease, such as exercising regularly and following the DASH diet. In fact, people who don't drink are usually pretty darn healthy. No need for you to get off the wagon now.

Watch Out! Alcohol & Meds

Alcohol can interfere with some types of high blood pressure medications. It can also increase the drugs' side effects, especially dizziness and depression. Pay attention to your body. If you are taking medications for your high blood pressure and notice you feel dizzy or depressed after having a drink, talk with your doctor. He or she will advise you about how much and when you can safely drink.

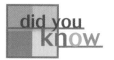

▶ *Americans get most of their caffeine—about 75 percent—from drinking coffee. The rest comes from tea (15 percent), soft drinks (10 percent), and chocolate (2 percent).*

The Caffeine Factor: What's the Buzz?

For many of us, starting a day without a cup of coffee or tea would be unthinkable—and perhaps undoable. It's not surprising, then, to know that caffeine is the world's most popular stimulant. Four out of five Americans guzzle it down in one form or another each day, usually to fight fatigue, boost concentration, or just to adjust their sights on a new day.

Whether or not consuming caffeine is good for our blood pressure—and our hearts—is a matter of hot debate. Scientists know that caffeine can cause a temporary spike in blood pressure, but does that mean it increases your risk for developing chronic high blood pressure? And if you already have high blood pressure, will cutting back on caffeine help you bring it down? Maybe. Maybe not.

When Only a Jolt Will Do

Caffeine raises blood pressure—temporarily at least—by constricting your blood vessels. Just how caffeine does this is not clear, although scientists think it may block the effects of a hormone called adenosine, which normally helps blood vessels stay open. (Adenosine also slows down brain activity, which is why caffeine temporarily makes you more alert.)

Studies have shown that drinking just one cup of coffee (a real measuring-cup cup, not a big, fat mug) raises both systolic and diastolic blood pressures by about 5 mm Hg each. The peak in pressure comes about 30 to 60 minutes after drinking the coffee and tends to dissipate about two hours after that.

Some studies have shown that people who consume caffeine regularly develop a tolerance to the stimulant. So if you tend to swig down four or five cups of coffee each morning, your blood pressure probably isn't going to be any higher than if you drank a single cup. (Caffeinated beverages also increase the excretion of calcium. If you drink a lot of coffee or cola, make sure you have an adequate calcium intake.)

The long-term buzz. Here's where the controversy starts. Studies that have looked at large populations of people and then compared the blood pressures of coffee drinkers with those of nondrinkers have been inconsistent. A few have shown a link between caffeine and high blood pressure, but most have not. In fact, one huge mega-analysis of 11 different studies from around the world (which included more than 143,000 individuals) found that coffee drinkers—even those who drank as much as six cups a day—were at no increased risk for developing either high blood pressure or heart disease.

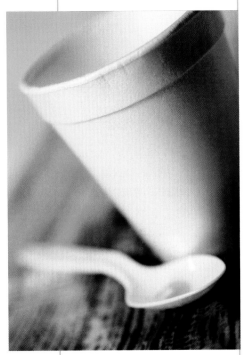

Some scientists think a better way to approach the issue, however, is to look at what happens to blood pressure after people quit drinking coffee. Researchers at the University of California at Berkeley designed such a study. They had 186 middle-aged coffee drinkers, all with normal blood pressure, drink the same brand of coffee for two months. The scientists then measured the men's blood pressure, both their resting pressure (taken while seated in a clinic) and their ambulatory, or "walking around," pressure (taken by a portable monitor at set intervals as the men followed their regular routines). Next, the men were split into three groups. One group continued to drink the same type and amount of coffee. A second group switched to decaffeinated coffee. The third group quit coffee altogether.

> **Pressure Point:** When cutting back, drink your coffee or soda from smaller cups so you don't feel deprived when drinking less.

The results, please. After two months, the men's blood pressures were measured again. The resting pressure taken in the clinic didn't change, but the ambulatory pressure of the men who either switched to decaf coffee or who didn't drink coffee at all dropped significantly: Systolic pressure fell an average of 3 mm Hg and diastolic pressure an average of 2 mm Hg.

(Remember: Even small drops in blood pressure can make a huge difference in your long-term health.)

Real-world pressures. The Berkeley study showed that it's important to measure caffeine's effect on blood pressure while people are going about their everyday activities. Caffeine researchers at Duke University Medical Center certainly agree with that observation. In one of their recent studies, they

Taking Tea to Heart

Tea is the most commonly consumed beverage in the world, second only to water. It may also—despite its caffeine—be one of the most healthful.

In recent years, scientists have gathered mounting evidence that both green and black teas, which are brewed from the leaves of the *Camellia sinensis* plant, protect against heart disease. (Herbal teas aren't included; they're made from other plants.)

Taking a tea rather than a coffee break may, therefore, be a smart decision for people who want to cut back, but not cut out, their daily dose of caffeine. Tea is a lot lighter on the caffeine. Eight ounces of black tea contain about 50 mg of caffeine; the same amount of green tea has about 30 mg. The same amount of brewed coffee, on the other hand, contains a hefty 135 mg.

hooked up 19 healthy people to portable monitors that checked blood pressure every 15 minutes for two days. On one day, the study's subjects were given caffeine pills equaling one cup of coffee; on another day they received pills that were the equivalent of four or five cups. On both days, they followed their normal routine. The result: The participants' blood pressure was an average of five points higher on the day they consumed the greater amount of caffeine.

So if you already have high blood pressure, you should take pause the next time you reach for your daily cup of joe.

Should You Hang Up Your Mug?

It depends on whom you ask. Most experts remain unconvinced that there is any strong link between caffeine and high blood pressure. In fact, a panel of experts from the National Heart, Lung, and Blood Institute stated flatly in 1997 that "no direct relationship between caffeine intake and elevated blood pressure has been found in most epidemiologic surveys."

Still, as a precaution (until the studies are more definitive), many doctors recommend that people with high blood pressure limit their caffeine to no more than 200 milligrams a day. That's about two 8-ounce cups of filtered coffee, four cups of tea, and four cans of caffeinated soda.

Of course, there are other solid health reasons for cutting back on caffeine:

> Too much caffeine can make you nervous and anxious and may interfere with your sleep.

> Caffeine can wreak havoc on your digestive system, causing heartburn, constipation, or diarrhea. It can also aggravate an existing stomach ulcer.

> Caffeine can irritate your bladder. Because it's a mild diuretic, it may also cause you to urinate more.

> Caffeine can be hard on your bones. Studies have shown that the more caffeine you consume, the more calcium you excrete in your urine. As a result, your bones may become thinner, less dense (a condition known as osteoporosis), putting you at greater risk for hip and other fractures as you age.

> If you're pregnant, consumption of caffeine may increase your risk of miscarrying or of delivering a baby that is underweight (less than five pounds).

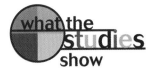

what the studies show

▶ *If you have high blood pressure, you should go easy on caffeine when you're under stress, say researchers from the University of Oklahoma Health Sciences Center Oklahoma City. In their study, the researchers gave 31 medical students—all coffee drinkers—either grapefruit juice spiked with caffeine or plain grapefruit juice. The stimulant sent the students' blood pressure up by as much as 5 mm Hg (systolic) and 4 mm Hg (diastolic). When the caffeine was combined with the stress of taking an exam, the student's blood pressure soared even higher, up to 10 and 6 points respectively.*

> **Pressure Point:** Caffeine is "hidden" in many over-the-counter medications, such as cold medicines, pain relievers, and appetite suppressants. If you want to avoid caffeine, read Rx labels carefully.

How to Back Away from Caffeine

Because caffeine is a mildly addictive drug, hanging up your coffee mug for good can result in several days of withdrawal symptoms—mostly headaches, fatigue, and irritability. Your best bet, therefore, is to do the deed gradually. Each day, halve the amount of caffeine you consume. If you drink eight cups of coffee a day, for example, cut back to four, then two, and so on. Do the same with caffeinated teas and sodas.

Here are some other tips for making the transition easier, especially if you have been using caffeine as a morning booster:

> To help you wake up, turn on the lights and open your window shades as soon as you get up in the morning.

> Exercise in the morning; it will give you a jolt of energy.

How Do You Brew Your Joe?

Before 1975, American men who drank five or more cups of coffee daily were two and a half times more likely to develop heart disease than their peers who shunned the stuff. Since 1975, however, men who drink that much coffee seem to have no greater risk for heart disease than those who never let java cross their lips.

What changed? Apparently, the way we brew our coffee. Around the mid-1970s, people started drinking filtered drip coffee rather than nonfiltered percolated (boiled) coffee. Some research indicates that drinking boiled coffee may raise cholesterol levels—and thus the risk for heart disease. The increased risk is due not to the caffeine in the coffee, but to oils in the coffee beans. When coffee is brewed through a paper filter, the oils are left behind.

Counting Caffeine

The caffeine content of beverages varies from product to product. Here are some averages to give you an idea of how much caffeine you're consuming each day. You won't find out this information from reading food labels; manufacturers are not required to list it on the label.

Source	How Much Caffeine
Coffee (8 oz. cup)	
Brewed, drip method	135 mg
Instant	95 mg
Decaffeinated	5 mg
Tea (8 oz. cup)	
Black tea (leaf or bag)	50 mg
Green tea	30 mg
Instant	15 mg
Caffeinated soft drinks (12 oz.)	
Colas	35 to 50 mg
Root beer	25 mg
Others	40 to 60 mg
Caffeinated waters (16.9 oz.)	50 to 125 mg
Chocolate (1.5 oz. bar)	10 to 30 mg
Over-the-counter headache medicines (2 tablets)	60 to 130 mg

> Make sure you eat some protein at breakfast. Research suggests that protein enhances brain alertness. Try low-fat yogurt or cottage cheese, or cereal with skim milk. Avoid fried protein foods, however, like bacon or sausages; the fat in these foods can leave you feeling out of it, plain lethargic.

> Some people become constipated for a few days after quitting coffee. Eating plenty of high-fiber foods (fruits, vegetables, and whole-grain breads and cereals) can help minimize this problem.

> If you get a temporary headache, take a pain reliever. Just make sure it contains no caffeine, or you'll simply be substituting one source of the stimulant for another.

7 Medication: A Consumer's Guide

Just 50 years ago a diagnosis of high blood

pressure was a death sentence. No longer.

Drugs have dramatically changed that discour-

aging picture. Medications can be life-savers,

but choosing the right one can be a daunting

task. Here is all the information you need to

make the right choice.

KEY CONCEPT

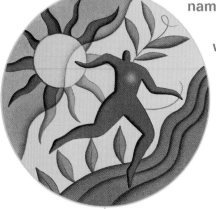

Rest assured, there is a drug out there with your name on it. The key is to find the one with maximum effectiveness and minimal side effects for you.

Your Blood Pressure on Drugs

Once your doctor gives a thumbs up to drug treatment to lower your high blood pressure, you have two jobs: Continue to embrace nondrug treatments—diet, exercise, stress reduction, and so forth—and be willing and able to work with your physician to limit the side effects and increase the effectiveness of the medication.

Medications to lower blood pressure are known as antihypertensives. These drugs can be extremely effective not only in reducing blood pressure but also in lowering the risk of future health problems, such as heart attacks and stroke. In fact, they might just save your life as they have done for a million or so others during the past two decades.

The drugs don't relieve symptoms, of course, because high blood pressure doesn't really have any symptoms. So it's not like taking an aspirin to relieve a pounding headache or an antibiotic to soothe a painful strep throat. Still, over time, your high blood pressure medication may make you feel better. In one study, people taking antihypertensives (five different kinds) reported having more energy, a happier mood, and all-round better health than people taking a placebo.

> **Pressure Point:** If you haven't been able to lower your blood pressure through lifestyle changes alone, don't take it as a personal failing. Scientists believe that genes often determine whether someone will need the help of medications to lower blood pressure.

The consequences. But high blood pressure drugs aren't miracle workers. They do have their side effects, of course, and some can be quite unpleasant—extreme fatigue, for example, and sexual problems. In rare cases, the side effects may even cancel out the drugs' considerable benefits. But despite what you may have heard about antihypertensives, the cure isn't worse than the ailment. Today there is a wider array of medications—nine different classes of drugs, in fact—than ever before for the treatment of high blood pressure. Each class of antihypertensives works on a specific system within the body—and, as you would guess, has different side effects. In collaboration with your doctor, you should be able to find a drug (or perhaps a combination of drugs) that is both effective and problem-free for you.

Which Drug Is Right for You?

For many years, people with high blood pressure had only a handful of medications to choose from. Now there are some 59 individual drugs, and the number is growing—there are seven new classes of HBP medications currently at some stage of development.

Each lowers blood pressure in a different way. Some ease the pumping of your heart, others widen the blood vessels, and still others regulate the levels of fluid in the body. Certain classes of medications are poor choices for some patients. Older people with HBP may not respond well to beta blockers. The same goes for young athletes who need to monitor their heart rate. ACE inhibitors, on the other hand, should not be prescribed for pregnant women. Persons with angina and high blood pressure may be placed on beta blockers, unless they are African Americans or elderly, in which case calcium channel blockers are more appropriate (see *Different Drugs for Different Folks*, p. 205).

Doctor, I Have a Question

Don't passively accept a prescription from your doctor. Ask questions that will help you use the drug effectively. For example:

- Why am I taking this medicine—what is the ultimate goal?

- How long will I be on the drug—a week, a month, a year, the rest of my life?

- When should I take this drug?

- Should I take this drug with food? If not, how long should I wait before or after a meal before taking the drug?

- What are the side effects?

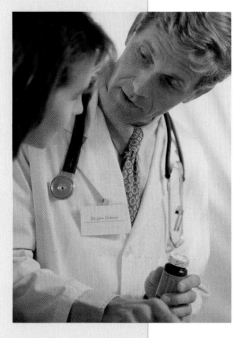

- Are there any prescription or over-the-counter medications that I should avoid taking while using this drug? (Be sure to give your doctor a complete list of medicines you currently use; include herbal supplements.)

- What should I do if I run out of the drug?

- What should I do if I forget to take a dose?

- Do you have any other special instructions for me?

On the next several pages, you will find a detailed rundown of every class of antihypertensive drug—everything from how they work to their troubling side effects. You should read this information even if lifestyle medicine—losing weight, exercising more, stopping smoking—is doing the trick of lowering your blood pressure. Some day you may need to take one of these medications. If you are already taking medication for your condition, then pay attention to details you might have overlooked—and have family members bone up on the medications as well so they can recognize potentially serious side effects quickly and seek emergency help.

Diuretics: The First Choice

Introduced in the 1950s, diuretics were among the first medications used to treat high blood pressure. They are the most commonly prescribed, partly because they have been found to be very effective for many people and partly because they cost much less than some of the newer antihypertensive drugs. In fact, if you are newly diagnosed with Stage 1 high blood pressure, this may be the first drug your doctor prescribes. Many studies indicate that 80 percent of patients with high blood pressure can be treated successfully with these drugs. African Americans, women, and the elderly tend to do well on diruetics.

> **Pressure Point:** Several studies have found that long-term exposure to diuretics can cause an increase in bone density and an overall reduction in hip fractures.

How they work. You may have heard diuretics referred to as "water pills." That's because they cause your kidneys to remove higher-than-normal amounts of sodium and water from your body. As a result, your body produces more urine. This is good for your blood pressure, because the less fluid in your body, the lower your blood pressure.

Diuretics work in a complex system of tiny tubes in the kidneys, known as nephrons, which regulate the balance of water and minerals, including salt. Each class of diuretics—thiazide, loop, and potassium-sparing—works in a different part of the tubes.

what the studies show

▶ *Among people with high blood pressure, taking a low daily dose of aspirin (75 milligrams) can reduce the risk for heart attack a dramatic 36 percent. But aspirin can also interfere with some blood pressure medications. So if you are already taking antihypertensives, talk with your doctor before taking aspirin regularly.*

CAUTION

While you are taking any antihypertensive drug, avoid alcohol, other medications taken without a doctor's permission, strenuous exercise, or a diet too low in salt—unless your doctor has advised it.

Thiazides

These are the most commonly prescribed type of diuretics, for several good reasons. They are relatively inexpensive; they can often be taken in small, one-a-day doses; and, perhaps, most importantly, they have proved effective not only in lowering blood pressure but also in preventing heart attack and stroke.

Thiazides work in one section of the far end, or distal, part of the nephrons, where large amounts of water and sodium are absorbed back into the body's bloodstream. Thiazides block this reabsorption, causing more fluid to be excreted in the urine. Scientists also believe that thiazides may relax muscles in the walls of blood vessels, enabling blood to flow more easily.

Thiazides are usually prescribed in low doses of 12.5 to 25 milligrams per day. Higher doses of these drugs (50 to 100 milligrams per day) have been found in some studies to increase the risk for heart attacks. Follow your doctor's instructions carefully when taking your medication.

You should know that thiazides can elevate total cholesterol, LDL cholesterol, and reduce HDL ("good") cholesterol. It is wise to have a blood test before starting the medicine and at periodic intervals to make sure that the drug is not having an adverse effect upon your blood fats.

Drug Wars: Diuretics and Other Meds

If your doctor plans to put you on a diuretic, it is important for you to ask her if any of the other medications you are currently taking might decrease the ability of the diuretic to lower your BP. Two common classes of medications used by people with arthritis or rheumatological problems do in fact decrease the overall effectiveness of diuretics: nonsteroidal anti-inflammatory drugs (NSAIDs), such as ibuprofen, and steroids.

This doesn't mean that your doctor should avoid trying a diuretic if you are on one of these medications; it just means that it might not work as well.

Loop

These diuretics block the reabsorption of sodium in an area of the nephron called the Loop of Henle. They are more powerful than thiazides and produce a more rapid formation of urine and a larger volume of urine output. Your doctor may recommend loop diuretics if thiazides haven't worked for you or if you have another condition, such as congestive heart failure, that causes your body to retain fluid.

Potassium-sparing

Unfortunately, in addition to getting rid of sodium, thiazide and loop diuretics cause the kidneys to flush potassium and other important minerals from the body. (If you are taking a diuretic, your doctor should carefully monitor its effects to be sure that your level of potassium, which passes out of the body with urine, is sufficient.) When your body's reserves of these minerals, especially potassium, gets too low, you can experience a range of problems, from weakness and muscle cramps to an irregular heartbeat.

> ### CAUTION
>
> **If you have kidney disease, you should avoid potassium-sparing diuretics. They can cause too-high levels of potassium, which may lead to heart irregularities and other problems.**

As their name suggests, potassium-sparing diuretics help rid your body of salt and fluids, but not potassium. Like thiazides, they work in a distal part of the nephron. Potassium-sparing diuretics, however, are less potent than thiazide or loop diuretics and can cause high blood potassium levels, so they are usually prescribed in combination with thiazides. When taking a potassium-sparing type of diuretic, avoid using a potassium-based salt substitute on your food. This could lead to a dangerous overload of the mineral.

> **Pressure Point:** Be patient when taking HBP medications. Although antihypertensive drugs will eventually lower BP, it could take a year to find one that works well for you with minimal side effects.

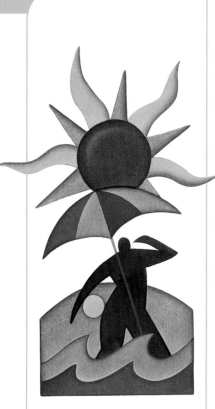

Side effects. The main side effect of diuretics is, not surprisingly, increased urination. Of course, this is a good side effect because it means the drug is doing its job and ridding the body of fluids (and thus lowering your blood pressure). But diuretics have some unwanted side effects, including weakness and fatigue; dizziness on standing (especially among older people); impotence; increased sensitivity to sunlight, possibly resulting in severe sunburn, redness, itching, or discoloration of skin or a change in vision; gout (a painful joint disorder triggered by excessive amounts of uric acid in the blood); a small increase in blood sugar and/or blood cholesterol levels; and dehydration. Contact your doctor if these symptoms persist or become bothersome or severe.

Watch Out! Taking Diuretics

○ Take diuretics in the morning; doing so will save you a trip or two to the bathroom in the middle of the night.

○ If diuretics upset your stomach, take them with food or milk.

○ Limit the amount of time you spend in direct sunlight; when out in the sun, be sure to use a sunscreen with SPF 15 or more and wear protective sunglasses.

○ Many diuretics (except for ethacrynic acid) contain sulfa, so persons allergic to sulfa should not take these drugs.

○ NSAIDs such as ibuprofen and steroids decrease the effectiveness of diuretics. If you take these drugs for arthritis or another problem, be sure to tell your doctor.

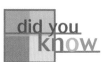

▶ *The International Olympic Committee has banned the use of beta blockers during their sports competitions because the drugs "can provide an advantage when concentration and nerves are vital, such as in archery and shooting."*

Beta Blockers: Heart Savers

Like diuretics, beta blockers have been used for decades to treat high blood pressure. They were first developed, however, to treat angina—recurring chest pain caused by blockages in the arteries that reduce blood flow to the heart. Only later did doctors discover, much to their delight, that beta blockers also lower blood pressure.

How they work. Beta blockers help the heart (and cause blood pressure to fall) because of their effect on structures within the cells of the heart and blood vessels known as beta adrenergic receptors. When stimulated by the stress hormones epinephrine and norepinephrine, these receptors cause blood vessels to constrict and the heart to beat faster and harder. Beta blockers (as their name implies) interfere with this process by binding to the receptor sites and preventing the hormones from affecting the heart. This type of drug also reduces the release of the hormone renin, which can elevate blood pressure.

Beta blockers are especially helpful for people with high blood pressure who have another heart condition, such as angina or arrhythmia (an irregular heartbeat). In addition, these drugs are frequently recommended for people with high blood pressure who have already had a heart attack. Beta blockers have been shown to lower the risk of having a second heart attack—by 40 percent, according to one study.

> **Pressure Point:** Beta blockers are also used to treat glaucoma, migraines, and some kinds of tremors. They also can help people overcome social phobias and other kinds of anxiety.

A select group. Not everyone can partake of beta blockers' benefits. Because these drugs cause the heart to beat less forcefully and at a slower rate, they are dangerous for people with congestive heart failure. Beta blockers also slightly constrict the airways in the lungs, so they are usually not prescribed for people with asthma or emphysema. (Good news, though, for asthmatics: In recent years, certain beta blockers, called beta-1-selective drugs, that "select out" receptors in the heart and blood vessels have hit the market; these drugs have little effect on the lungs. These selective beta blockers seem to have a less adverse effect on cholesterol and blood sugar than nonselective versions.)

Because beta blockers lower the body's response to epinephrine, these drugs can mask the warning signs of lower blood sugar levels—a potentially dangerous situation for people with diabetes. Persons who suffer from depression should not be placed on beta blockers because the drugs can worsen the condition.

Side effects. Fatigue is the most common side effect of beta

what the studies show

▶ *Taking beta blockers for high blood pressure increases your risk for developing diabetes by 28 percent, according to a study by researchers at Johns Hopkins University School of Medicine in Baltimore. If you are taking beta blockers and are overweight or have a family history of diabetes, you should ask your doctor whether other medicines may be just as effective for treating your high blood pressure.*

blockers. If you enjoy sports and other physical activities, these drugs may not be the right choice for you. Ask your doctor how intensely you can exercise while on the drug. Some people may also experience dizziness, especially on rising. (Changing positions slowly when sitting and/or standing up may help decrease the dizziness). Other possible side effecs include wheezing (in people whose lungs are sensitive to allergens and irritants or who have lung disease); reduced sex drive (in men and women); impotence; difficulty sleeping or vivid, sometimes nightmarish, dreams; heartburn, diarrhea, constipation, or gas; cold hands and feet (especially in older people); weight gain. Beta blockers can also elevate triglyceride and blood sugar levels.

The side effects of these drugs are usually temporary. Contact your doctor if the effects persist or become bothersome or severe.

> ### Watch Out! Taking Beta Blockers
>
> ○ Take the drugs with meals or soon after eating. Food slows down the drugs' absorption and helps reduce side effects.
>
> ○ Take and record your pulse daily to be sure it doesn't drop too low. Ask your doctor what a too-low pulse would be for you. If your pulse falls to that level, call your doctor to see if you should take your medication that day.
>
> ○ Never stop taking these drugs without consulting with your doctor. Beta blockers have a powerful effect on the heart; an abrupt stoppage of the drugs could be dangerous.

ACE Inhibitors: Growing in Popularity

Unlike diuretics or beta blockers, ACE (angiotensin-converting enzyme) inhibitors don't produce fatigue, which is one of the main reasons this class of drugs has become so popular in recent years for the treatment of high blood pressure. These medications work best in persons who produce high levels of the hormone renin—a condition called high-renin hypertension. The dosages of these drugs vary greatly depending on the severity of your high blood pressure and the presence of other medical problems.

How they work. ACE inhibitors lower blood pressure by interfering with an enzyme—renin—that converts angiotensin I into angiotensin II, a powerful hormone that causes blood vessels to constrict and blood pressure to rise. Angiotensin II also stimulates the release of aldosterone, a hormone that causes the body to hold on to water and salt, increasing blood pressure levels even more. ACE inhibitors also prevent the breakdown of bradykinin, a substance in the blood that dilates blood vessels and leads to a reduction in BP.

> **Pressure Point:** Although ACE inhibitors are expensive, one study showed that they decreased the risk of death and reduced hospital visits, saving more than $1,500 per patient over three years.

ACE inhibitors appear to have fewer side effects than other drugs for high blood pressure, but they are not recommended for everyone. If you have severe kidney disease, for example, you should probably not take these drugs because they can lead to kidney failure. In addition, a recent study found that ACE inhibitors cause the kidney to retain potassium, which can result in heart problems if levels become too high.

If you are a woman who is pregnant or even thinking about getting pregnant, you should also avoid these drugs; they can cause babies to be born with dangerously low blood pressure, kidney failure, and other serious health problems.

On the other hand, ACE inhibitors, unlike diuretics and beta blockers, don't raise blood cholesterol, which makes them a good antihypertensive medication for people with high cholesterol. This class of drugs is also a logical first choice for diabetics with high blood pressure. ACE inhibitors improve a person's ability to respond to insulin and protect a diabetic from kidney damage.

Side effects. About 25 percent of people taking ACE inhibitors develop a persistent dry cough. Women are three times more likely than men to experience this side effect. And here's an ironic twist: The problem is worse for nonsmokers than for smokers. (Sorry, you still need to give up your ciga-

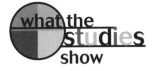

what the studies show

▶ *ACE inhibitors and thiazide diuretics are a strong one-two punch for lowering blood pressure. Some studies have shown, however, that switching to a low-salt diet can be just as effective as adding the diuretic. So if you want to minimize the medications you're taking (and their side effects), don't forget to cut back on the salt in your diet.*

▶ *People who take the ACE inhibitor ramipril have fewer heart attacks and strokes, according to findings published in 2000 by researchers for the HOPE (Heart Outcomes Prevention Evaluation) study. But that's not all: The people taking ramipril were also 30 percent less likely to develop diabetes.*

rettes.) Changing to another ACE inhibitor can sometimes help get rid of the cough, so talk to your doctor if you develop this side effect.

Less common side effects include skin rash; diminished sense of taste, and swelling of the mouth, tongue, and lips. Swelling usually starts with the first dose. Some experts recommend taking a dose of Benadryl or a steroid upon experiencing swelling. Talk with your doctor about this option.

> **Watch Out!** Taking ACE Inhibitors
>
> ⊃ Most ACE inhibitors can be taken with or without food. But some (such as captopril and moexipril) are best taken on an empty stomach one hour before meals. Follow your doctor's instructions.
>
> ⊃ Avoid the use of aspirin and other nonsteroidal anti-inflammatory drugs such as ibuprofen or naproxen. Use acetaminophen for pain relief.

Angiotensin II Receptor Blockers: Newer, Effective, Expensive

These drugs, which won FDA approval in 1995, are also referred to as AT I receptor blockers. The first of these to be approved was losartan, sold under the brand name Cozaar and in combination with a diuretic.

How they work. Like their first cousins, the ACE inhibitors, the AT I receptor blockers stop the hormone angiotensin II from doing its thing (constricting blood vessels). But instead of blocking the formation of angiotensin II, they prevent the hormone from hooking up with its receptor sites within the blood vessels. As a result, angiotensin II can't constrict the blood vessels, which means they remain open—lowering BP.

Angiotensin II receptor blockers have an advantage over ACE inhibitors: They don't make you cough. And one of the drugs, losartan, may also help you avoid the sexual dysfunction that sometimes accompanies other HBP medications. After 12 weeks of treatment with losartan, the percentage of men reporting impotence dropped from 75.3 to 11.1, according to a study conducted at Wake Forest University.

One of the biggest disadvantages of angiotensin II receptor blockers is that they are not available in generic form (and won't be for many years), which makes them an expensive choice for treating high blood pressure. Also, as with ACE inhibitors, women who are pregnant or who are even considering becoming pregnant should avoid these drugs. So should women who are breastfeeding.

Side effects. Angiotensin II receptor blockers appear to

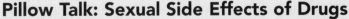

Pillow Talk: Sexual Side Effects of Drugs

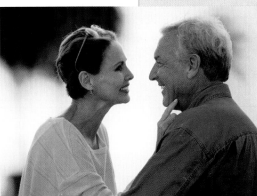

Antihypertensives have long been blamed for causing sexual problems in both men and women. Sexual problems, however, are primarily a result of the high blood pressure itself, not the drugs. High blood pressure damages and constricts small blood vessels in the sexual organs of both genders. Without proper blood flow, these organs are unable to function normally. Still, certain medications do exacerbate sexual dysfunction. What can you do to avoid unwanted sexual side effects?

- Talk openly and honestly with your doctor about your concerns and about any sexual problems you're experiencing—both before and after you start on your medication. You and your doctor can then make a more informed choice about the dose and type of medication that's best for you.

- Discuss with your doctor taking another medication to help restore sexual function, such as Viagra (sildenafil), the popular pill for male impotence.

have few side effects, although some people have reported that the drugs make them feel tired or dizzy. In rare cases, people also experience insomnia, diarrhea, indigestion, and a stuffy nose while taking these drugs. Contact your doctor if these symptoms persist or become bothersome or severe.

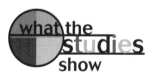

what the studies show

▶ *A recent study found that people who took either certain calcium channel blockers or diuretics experienced changes in brain tissue; those who took beta blockers had no such changes. If you find yourself experiencing unpleasant mental or emotional changes while taking an antihypertensive drug, consult your physician about changing medications.*

▶ *Could calcium channel blockers be the male version of the Pill? Possibly, say researchers from the New York University School of Medicine and the University of Rochester Medical Center in Rochester, New York. The drug appears to fatten the sperm with cholesterol, which leaves the sperm unable to fertilize an egg. Once men stop taking calcium channel blockers, their sperm is able to shed the cholesterol and become fertile again.*

Watch Out! Taking Angiotensin II Receptor Blockers

◐ You can take these drugs with or without food.

◐ To avoid a dangerously high buildup of potassium in your body, don't use salt substitutes containing potassium while taking these drugs.

Calcium Channel Blockers: Effective But Safe?

Available in the United States since the 1970s, calcium channel blockers (CCBs) have come under heavy fire in recent years. Some studies have shown that although they lower blood pressure, they may not decrease the risk of heart attack. As a result, these drugs—also known as calcium antagonists—usually are not prescribed as a first-choice treatment for high blood pressure, especially for people with congestive heart failure.

How they work. CCBs lower blood pressure by plugging up the entrances to tiny passages, called calcium channels, in the muscle cells that surround blood vessels. Calcium, which causes the muscle cells to contract, is then unable to enter the channels. Without the calcium and the contractions, the blood vessels remain dilated and blood pressure comes down. Some calcium channel blockers also work directly on the heart, slowing down the speed and force with which that mighty organ pumps. Again, blood pressure drops.

> **Pressure Point:** Calcium channel blockers do not interfere with the calcium your body uses to build bone.

Because fatigue is not a major side effect of calcium channel blockers, they are sometimes prescribed to people with active lifestyles. These drugs have also proven especially effective in African Americans and older people, as well as in people suffering from angina. What's more, NSAIDs don't reduce the effectiveness of CCBs the way they do other HBP drugs. If you have an irregular heartbeat (heart arrhythmia) or liver disease, however, you should use these drugs very cautiously.

Some calcium channel blockers are short-acting. They lower blood pressure quickly, sometimes within half an hour, but their effects last only a few hours. Long-acting versions of these

Calcium Channel Blockers: Two Thumbs Up?

Short-acting CCBs have been found to raise heart attack risk by 60 percent, which is why few doctors prescribe them today except in emergency situations. The safety of long-acting CCBs, on the other hand, remains hotly disputed. Two large studies have reached very different conclusions. One showed that long-acting CCBs increased heart attack risk by 27 percent. Another found that the long-acting drugs posed no problems at all.

Now what? The National Institutes of Health hopes to answer that question within a year when the results from an eight-year study will be reported. In the meantime, if you have been prescribed a calcium channel blocker for high blood pressure, discuss with your doctor why this is the best drug for you. You and your doctor may decide to switch to a diuretic, a beta blocker, or an ACE inhibitor—equally beneficial drugs with better track records for protecting the heart.

drugs are absorbed into the body at a much slower pace, and they stay active much longer.

Side effects. People seem to tolerate calcium channel blockers quite well, which is one reason they became quickly popular after they were first introduced. Some people, however, do experience constipation while taking these drugs. Studies show that postmenopausal women who take short-acting CCBs have twice the risk of developing breast cancer than other women. Also, in another study, it was shown that people taking CCBs were twice as likely to be hospitalized for bleeding in the gastrointestinal (GI) tract as people taking beta blockers.

Other possible side effects include headache; a rapid heartbeat; dizziness (changing positions slowly when sitting and/or standing up may help decrease the dizziness); nausea; and swelling, especially of the gums, lower legs, and ankles.

Watch Out! Taking Calcium Channel Blockers

◐ Avoid grapefruit or grapefruit juice. A substance in grapefruit appears to interfere with the liver's ability to clear some calcium channel blockers from the body. As a result, the drugs may linger in your bloodstream—perhaps building up to toxic levels.

◐ Taking calcium channel blockers with a high-fat meal can sometimes speed up—perhaps dangerously so—their effect on your body. Ask your doctor if you should avoid taking your medication with high-fat foods.

◐ Constipation may be relieved by drinking more water, eating foods that are high in fiber (vegetables, fruits, bran), and exercising.

◐ Avoid becoming dehydrated or overheated. Avoid saunas, strenuous exercise in hot weather, and alcoholic beverages. Drink plenty of fluids.

Alpha Blockers: Two Birds with One Stone?

Since people with high blood pressure also suffer from high blood cholesterol and, as a result, have a higher risk for heart attack, wouldn't it be a godsend to have a drug that lowered both. Perhaps there is such a drug—the alpha blocker.

How they work. In addition to beta receptors, humans have nodes called alpha blockers. When stimulated by epinephrine or norepinephrine, the nodes cause blood vessels to narrow. Alpha blockers seem to prevent the alpha receptor from binding with the hormones epinephrine and norepinephrine in the walls of your blood vessels (particularly your smaller arteries). Without that hormonal hookup, your blood vessels stay relaxed and open, increasing blood flow.

Alpha blockers seem to lower cholesterol and triglycerides, so if you have high blood pressure and high cholesterol (especially high LDL cholesterol—the kind that clogs arteries), these drugs may be doubly beneficial. Alpha blockers may also be a good choice for older men with high blood pressure who have a prostate problem known as benign prostatic hypertrophy (BPH). The drugs have been shown to ease some of the urination difficulties associated with BPH, including the frequent need to go to the bathroom at night.

Different Drugs for Different Folks

If you are . . .	You May Prefer	You May Not Prefer
Over the age of 50	Alpha blockers; beta blockers; ACE inhibitors	None
Over the age of 65	Thiazide diuretics; ACE inhibitors; calcium channel blockers	Central alpha agonists
African American	Thiazide diuretics; ACE inhibitors	Beta blockers
White	Beta blockers; ACE inhibitors	None
Physically active	ACE inhibitors; calcium channel blockers; alpha blockers	Beta blockers
Pregnant	Methyldopa (a central alpha agonist)	ACE inhibitors; angiotensin II receptor blockers
If you have...		
Diabetes	ACE inhibitors; low-dose thiazide diuretics; central alpha agonists; alpha blockers	High-dose thiazide diuretics; beta blockers
Congestive heart failure	ACE inhibitors; thiazide diuretics	Beta blockers (except carvedilol); calcium channel blockers (except amlodipine)
Heart disease	Beta blockers	Blood vessel dilators
A history of heart attack	Beta blockers; ACE inhibitors	None
Angina	Beta blockers; calcium channel blockers; alpha blockers	None
High cholesterol	ACE inhibitors; calcium channel blockers; alpha blockers	High-dose diuretics; beta blockers
Kidney problems	Loop diuretics; ACE inhibitors; minoxidil (a blood vessel dilator)	Potassium-sparing diuretics
Osteoporosis	Thiazide diuretics	None
High triglycerides	Alpha blockers	High-dose thiazide diuretics; beta blockers
Asthma	None	Beta blockers
Hyperthyroidism	Beta blockers	None
An enlarged prostate gland (also known as BPH)	Alpha blockers	None
Migraine headaches	Certain beta blockers and calcium channel blockers	None
History of depression	None	Central alpha agonists; beta blockers; reserpine (a peripheral-acting adrenergic antagonist)

But there is a new concern about alpha blockers. In 2000, researchers at the National Heart, Lung, and Blood Institute halted one part of a large, ongoing study of blood pressure medications because their data showed that the alpha blocker doxazosin actually increased the risk for heart attacks and heart failure. The researchers advised people taking alpha blockers to consult with their doctors about a possible alternative.

Side effects. When you take alpha blockers for the first time you may feel light-headed, particularly as you stand up from a sitting or lying position. You may even faint. This is because alpha blockers can cause blood pressure to drop quickly (a condition called orthostatic hypotension). To help you avoid this problem (called a first-dose effect), your doctor will start you off with a very small dose of the drug and then slowly increase the dosage as your body adjusts to the drug's effects.

Other possible side effects include headaches, a rapid heart-beat, and nausea. Also, be aware that alpha blockers can lose their effectiveness the longer you use them. This is because your body responds to the lower blood pressure by holding on to more salt and water. Taking a diuretic along with the alpha blocker usually solves the problem. If any side effect persists or becomes bothersome or severe, contact your doctor.

Watch Out! Taking Alpha Blockers

○ Avoid driving for 12 to 24 hours after taking your first dose of an alpha blocker or after the dosage is increased.

○ To avoid dizziness, rise slowly when standing.

○ Take the medication at night before going to bed, but be careful of dizziness when getting out of bed for a trip to the bathroom.

Central Alpha Agonists: Fiddling with Your Brain

These drugs work directly on the brain rather than on the blood vessels. They prevent the brain from sending nerve impulses that normally signal the arteries to narrow and the heart to speed up its pumping action.

Because of their potentially strong side effects—especially dizziness and drowsiness—central alpha agonists aren't prescribed as often as they used to be. You will be given these only after other drugs have failed to lower your blood pressure. Under certain circumstances, however, central alpha agonists are still useful—for people who have migraine headaches or frequent panic attacks, for example, or for those who are going through drug or alcohol withdrawal. The drugs sometimes help reduce symptoms associated with these conditions.

One central alpha agonist, clonidine, is now available in an easy-to-use patch that you apply to your skin once a week. (These patches are similar to the nicotine ones that people use to stop smoking.) Another one of these drugs, methyldopa, is considered a first-choice drug for pregnant women with high blood pressure because it has been shown to be safe for unborn babies. Methyldopa is available in both pill and liquid forms.

Side effects. In addition to dizziness and drowsiness, possible side effects include nausea, rapid heartbeat, headache, dry mouth, constipation, fatigue and sleep problems, depression and anxiety, and impotence. Contact your doctor if these symptoms persist or become severe.

Watch Out! Taking Central Alpha Agonists

○ These drugs can make you drowsy. Don't drive until you know how your drug affects you.

○ If you are taking the liquid form of methyldopa, be sure to shake it well before using it.

○ Dispose of used clonidine patches carefully. A discarded patch will still contain enough medication to be harmful to children or pets.

○ Stopping use of these drugs can cause your blood pressure to rise quickly to dangerous levels. Never go off these drugs without talking with your doctor.

Peripheral-Acting Adrenergic Antagonists: Potent Medicine

These drugs don't work on the brain, but on another—or peripheral—area of the nervous system, where they interfere with the workings of the hormones epinephrine and norepinephrine. Of the three drugs currently available in this class, two (guanadrel and guanethidine) block nerve cells from releasing the hormones, while a third (reserpine) prevents the hormones from reaching their intended destinations in the body, making it impossible for the substances to tighten and narrow blood vessels.

Peripheral-acting adrenergic antagonists are quite potent. Guanadrel and guanethidine can cause your blood pressure to quickly plunge when you stand up or when you're exercising. The drop in pressure may be fast and hard enough to make you faint. Reserpine has been linked to the sudden onset of serious depression. For these reasons, peripheral-acting adrenergic antagonists are usually prescribed only in severe cases of high blood pressure that haven't responded well to other medications. To help offset some of their side effects, peripheral-acting adrenergic antagonists are often combined with other antihypertensives, such as diuretics, with great success.

> **Pressure Point:** Most people with high blood pressure forget to take at least one dose of their medication a week.

Side effects. In addition to dizziness and depression, possible side effects of these drugs include drowsiness, diarrhea, dry mouth, stuffy nose, loss of appetite, nausea, nasal congestion, and impotence. Contact your doctor if these symptoms persist or become bothersome or severe.

Watch Out! Taking Peripheral-Acting Adrenergic Antagonists

- ◑ Avoid standing for long periods of time, particularly if out in the sun.
- ◑ Take your time when rising from bed in the morning.
- ◑ If you experience insomnia or nightmares or become depressed while taking these drugs, contact your doctor right away.

Blood Vessel Dilators: A Last Resort

Because of their serious side effects in some people, blood vessel dilators are usually reserved for persons with severe hypertension whose BP has been unresponsive to other medications.

How they work. Blood vessel dilators work directly on the muscular walls of the small arteries, relaxing them and opening them up so blood can flow smoothly and unimpeded. They are among the most powerful antihypertensives, with potent side effects.

Side effects. It's common for blood vessel dilators to speed up the heart and cause the body to retain water—two developments that can quickly raise rather than lower blood pressure. That's why your doctor will almost certainly prescribe a beta blocker (to slow down your heartbeat) and a diuretic (to rid your body of fluids) along with the blood vessel dilator.

Other possible side effects include flushing (feeling of warmth), dizziness, headache, loss of appetite, gastrointestinal problems, eye tearing, stuffy nose, skin rash, and breast tenderness. One blood vessel dilator, minoxidil, may cause your body hair to grow in thicker or darker; the other, hydralazine, may increase your risk for lupus, an inflammatory disease in which the body attacks its own cells and tissue.

> **CAUTION**
>
> Minoxidil, a blood vessel dilator, can worsen angina (chest pain) or cause other heart problems. If you experience any kind of pain or discomfort in your chest while taking this medication (or at any other time), call your doctor immediately or seek other medical help.

Watch Out! Taking Blood Vessel Dilators

- Keep all appointments with your doctor. He or she will want to monitor your heart carefully while you're taking these drugs.
- These drugs can make you drowsy. Don't drive until you know how your drug affects you.

Combination Drugs: Doubly Effective

If you have Stage 1 or Stage 2 high blood pressure, you have a 50-50 chance of needing only a single drug to control your high blood pressure. But if that first drug doesn't work, your doctor may opt to add a second drug to your treatment. Diuretics are often combined with beta blockers, ACE inhibitors, or angiotensin II receptor blockers, for example. Other common combos are calcium channel blockers and ACE inhibitors.

Combination drugs can be more effective than single drugs, and because they use smaller doses of each medication, they can also produce fewer side effects. Often, the two drugs are mixed together into a single pill or capsule, which makes taking the medications very easy (see the next page).

Winning Combinations

Two different drugs for high blood pressure are often blended together into a single pill. Here are some examples.

Generic Combinations	Brand Name
Beta blockers and diuretics	
Atenolol (50 or 100 mg) & chlorthalidone (25 mg)	Tenoretic
Bisoprolol fumarate (2.5, 5, or 10 mg)& hydrochlorothiazide (6.25 mg)	Ziac
Metoprolol tartrate (50 or 100 mg) & hydrochlorothiazide (25 or 50 mg)	Lopressor HCT
Nadolol (40 or 80 mg) & bendroflumerthiazide (5 mg)	Corzide
Propranolol hydrochloride (40 or 80 mg) & hydrochlorothiazide (25 mg)	Inderide
Propranolol hydrochloride (extended release) (80, 120, or 160 mg) & hydrochlorothiazide (50 mg)	Inderide LA
Timolol maleate (10 mg) & hydrochlorothiazide (25 mg)	Timolide
ACE inhibitors and diuretics	
Benazepril hydrochloride (5, 10, or 20 mg) & hydrochlorothiazide (6.25, 12.5, or 25 mg)	Lotensin HCT
Captopril (25 or 50 mg) & hydrochlorothiazide (15 or 25 mg)	Capozide
Enalapril maleate (5 or 10 mg) & hydrochlorothiazide (12.5 or 25 mg)	Vaseretic
Lisinopril (10 or 20 mg) & hydrochlorothiazide (12.5 or 25 mg)	Prinzide, Zestoretic
Angiotensin II receptor blockers and diuretics	
Losartan potassium (50 mg) & hydrochlorothiazide (12.5 mg)	Hyzaar
Calcium antagonists and ACE inhibitors	
Amlodipine besylate (2.5 or 5 mg) & benazepril hydrochloride (10 or 20 mg)	Lotrel
Diltiazem hydrochloride (180 mg) & enalapril maleate (5 mg)	Teczem
Verapamil hydrochloride (extended release (180 or 240 mg) & trandolapril (1, 2, or 4 mg)	Tarka
Felodipine (5 mg) & enalapril maleate (5 mg)	Lexxel
Diuretics and diuretics	
Triamterene (37.5, 50, or 75 mg) & hydrochlorothiazide (25 or 50 mg)	Dyazide, Maxide
Spironolactone (25 or 50 mg) & hydrochlorothiazide (25 or 50 mg)	Aldactazide
Amiloride hydrochloride (5 mg) and hydrochlorothiazide (50 mg)	Moduretic

SOURCE: The Sixth Report of the Joint National Committee on Prevention, Detection, Evaluation, and Treatment of High Blood Pressure

Help in a Hurry

Sometimes blood pressure reaches dangerous levels and must be brought down right away to avoid a heart attack, stroke, or other serious health problems. In these cases, an antihypertensive (usually a blood vessel dilator or an alpha or beta blocker) will be injected directly into a vein. The goal is usually to reach a blood pressure reading of at least 160/100. The numbers are brought down gradually, however, over a period of hours, not minutes; pressure that falls too fast can result in too little blood reaching the heart, brain, and other organs.

> **Pressure Point:** Half of the people who take antihypertensives need only one drug to lower their blood pressure to healthy levels. Another 30 percent do it with a combination of two drugs.

Several combination drugs have been approved by the Food and Drug Administration as first-choice treatments for high blood pressure. They include Ziac, a mixture of the diuretic hydrochlorothiazide and the beta blocker bisoprolol fumarate, and Capozide, which combines hydrochlorothiazide with the ACE inhibitor captopril. Side effects—mostly drowsiness and sun sensitivity—of these combos tend to be mild and temporary.

The Problems with Pills: How to Avoid Them

All drugs have potential side effects, and antihypertensives are no exception. But not all medications for high blood pressure affect everybody in the same way. You won't really know if you'll have a problem with a particular drug until you take it. And if you do suffer side effects, you don't have to live with them.

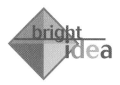

▶ *The decrease in blood pressure triggered by antihypertensive medications can cause blood to flow rapidly from your head to other parts of your body. Dizziness can result. If you are taking medications and suddenly find yourself feeling weak, faint, and possibly nauseated to the point of vomiting, lie down at once with your feet at a level higher than your head. Such action will help return blood to your head. If this doesn't help, you will need emergency medical care.*

Talk with your doctor. Let him or her know what you're experiencing. There are other medication choices out there—including one that will be just right for you. But remember: only physicians, physician assistants, nurse practitioners, and other health professionals are authorized to prescribe drugs and to make dosage adjustments. Changing or stopping any prescribed medication on the advice of a friend or other nonmedical provider can be very dangerous and, in extreme cases, may prove fatal.

Your Drug Protocol: What to Expect

The first choice of medication for uncomplicated cases of hypertension is usually either a diuretic or a beta blocker. These drugs have been around the longest, so volumes are known about their safety and effectiveness. They also tend to be less expensive. Your doctor will probably start you on a low dose of the drug, which may be gradually increased if your blood pressure doesn't respond.

If the medication doesn't rein in your blood pressure within a reasonable time or if it creates troublesome side effects, your doctor may prescribe one of the other classes of antihypertensives. Or you may be put on two or even more drugs from different classes. Many of the drug classes team up to lower blood pressure, often canceling out each other's side effects.

When the pressure is too great. If you have a severe case of high blood pressure, the first drug you receive may be a central alpha agonist or a blood vessel dilator; both will lower your blood pressure quickly. If your doctor believes your blood pressure is dangerously high (putting you in imminent risk of a heart attack, for example), you may be admitted into a hospital so you can be carefully watched as your blood pressure is brought down. (See *Help in a Hurry*, on p. 211.)

Staying the Course

Your doctor should ask you to return one to two months after you start your medication to see if the treatment is working and what, if any, side effects you may be experiencing. Of course, you may be asked to see your doctor sooner if you have Stage 2 or Stage 3 high blood pressure or another major health condition, such as diabetes or heart disease, or if you call the doctor to report a particularly persistent or troubling problem with the medication, such as debilitating fatigue or headaches.

During these checkups your blood pressure will be taken at least twice. You'll also be given a general physical examination and some routine laboratory tests, such as a blood test to see if and how the medication is altering your body chemistry (such as your sodium and potassium levels), and a urine test to check how well your kidneys are functioning.

CAUTION

Before any surgery or dental work, tell your physician or dentist that you are taking high blood pressure medications.

> **Pressure Point:** Half of Americans with high blood pressure fail to keep regularly scheduled appointments with their doctor—one of the major reasons the blood pressure of so many people is out of control.

Speak up. Your job during each checkup is to share your observations with your doctor about how the medication is affecting you. Also, tell your doctor about how you're progressing with your attempts to adopt a healthier lifestyle. Be honest. Only with all the facts in hand can you and your doctor decide whether to continue with your current treatment plan or to start devising a new one.

Once your blood pressure is under control, follow-up doctor visits are usually scheduled every three to six months. But never hesitate to call or visit your doctor with your questions or concerns. You have the right to be in charge of decisions affecting your health. And your doctor has the responsibility to provide you with accurate information about your condition and to allow you to actively participate in your care.

Less May Be More

Once your blood pressure has been under control for at least a year, you should talk with your doctor about beginning a "step down" treatment—a gradual reduction of either the number of drugs that you're taking or their dosages—or perhaps both. The goal is to find the minimum amount of medication necessary to maintain your blood pressure at an acceptable level. Not everybody is able to step down from their medications. Your chances of successfully doing it are greatest if you've also made lifestyle changes, like controlling your weight, quitting smoking, eating well, limiting sodium levels, and staying active.

Ditching drugs altogether. Some lucky people—mostly those with Stage 1 blood pressure—are able to discontinue their medications altogether. If your doctor does allow you to discontinue medication, you need to stay vigilant to avoid slipping back into old, unhealthful habits. Blood pressure usually creeps back up, sometimes months or years after stopping

Helpful Herbs: Garlic and Hawthorn

A pungent pressure-reducer. Since the Stone Age, garlic (*Allium sativum*) has been used as a medicinal herb. In ancient Egypt, workers on the pyramids rioted when the herb, which they believed kept them strong and healthy, was omitted from their daily food rations.

In recent times, scientists have found evidence suggesting that eating garlic daily may reduce the risk for heart disease, perhaps by lowering blood pressure and keeping sticky platelets from clogging arteries. Fresh garlic is the most potent form of the herb. To maintain low blood pressure, herbalists recommend taking 1 to 3 cloves of garlic each day. Sound unappealing? You can try garlic capsules instead; read labels for recommended dosages.

Healing hawthorn. A thorny shrub used as a living fence throughout much of Europe, hawthorn (*Crataegus laebvigata*) has long been recognized for its heart-healthy properties. Herbalists prescribe the herb as a mild heart tonic. It is also thought to lower blood pressure by dilating the blood vessels.

You can take hawthorn in tincture form (10 to 20 drops three times a day) or in pill form (300 to 450 milligrams a day). You can also make hawthorn tea. Steep the dried flowers and berries in hot water for 10 to 15 minutes; drink two to three times a day.

Warning: If you have a heart condition, are pregnant, or are taking any kind of medications, be sure to talk with your doctor before using hawthorn.

medication, especially when people fail to stay committed to a healthier lifestyle. Be sure to continue to see your doctor regularly to have your blood pressure checked. And continue to watch your weight, walk those three miles every day, cook those low-fat meals (without salt!), practice your favorite stress-reducing strategies, and do all those other daily actions that help you maintain a healthy blood pressure.

> ➤ **Pressure Point:** Make up a list of all your prescriptions and store it in your wallet or someplace where it can be found in case of an emergency.

Minding Your Meds

Because high blood pressure is a "silent" condition, without any visible symptoms, it can be easy to forget to take your medications. You might even consider it okay to take a break from your medication—when you're on vacation, for instance.

Don't fool yourself. Just because you continue to feel physically fine when you skip or stop your high blood pressure medication doesn't mean you're not putting your health in jeopardy. In fact, going off your meds suddenly can be downright dangerous. One of the most common reasons why blood pressure drugs fail to work is that patients fail to take them as prescribed (called noncompliance). Most high blood pressure experts will tell you that, for the most part, there is no such thing as unmanageable hypertension, only unmanageable patients.

You need to take your medications as prescribed. Here are some tips to help you do just that.

Get into a rut. Place your pills next to some object that you use every day, like your toothbrush or eyeglasses. Many single-dose antihypertensives are best taken with the morning meal, so you may want to keep them in the kitchen near your breakfast things. Medications that are to be taken right before bed can be placed on your nightstand, so you won't go to sleep without seeing them. (Make sure, however, that all medications are out of reach of children and pets.)

Get alarmed. Set an alarm clock or a watch with a built-in alarm to remind you of when it's time to take your medication.

Find a nag. Ask someone close to you to remind you to take your medications—at least until the habit becomes part of your daily routine. If you live alone, a friend or relative could call you at prearranged times.

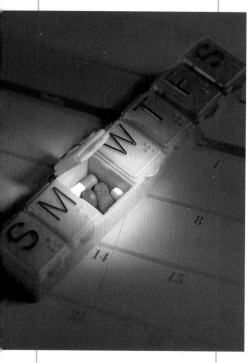

Use a pillbox. If you are taking more than one kind of medication, purchase an inexpensive plastic pillbox from your pharmacist. These handy containers come with compartments for each day of the week. Load them once a week with your medicines and you'll be able to keep track of which pills you take and when.

Go into the light. Don't reach for drugs at night in a dark bedroom. Always put on a light to make sure you don't take the wrong pill.

Get (and stick) with the program. Take your medication in the correct doses and at the right time of day. Your doctor (and the drug's label) will tell you what the dosage and timing should be. Taking a medication too early might release too much of the drug into your system and aggravate side effects. Taking it too late might cause your blood pressure to rise. If you are supposed to take your medication twice or more a day, do so at the hourly intervals indicated on the drug's label or by your doctor.

Don't change. Never change your dosage—either up or down—without talking with your doctor first. If for some reason you do forget to take your medication, call your doctor to see what you should do. Don't try to correct the error by doubling up the dosage the next time you're supposed to take it.

Keep track of any side effects. Share this information with your doctor at your next office visit—or sooner if the side effects are particularly bothersome.

Don't leave home without it. If you're traveling by plane, be sure to pack your medication in your carry-on luggage in its original container. That way, if your luggage is lost or your flight is delayed, you'll have your medication and its instructions with you.

> **Pressure Point:** According to the National Council on Patient Information and Education, almost two-thirds of people prescribed medicine to control high blood pressure stop taking it (against their doctor's advice) within three years.

When Medications Don't Mix

Many prescription and over-the-counter drugs can interfere with certain blood pressure medications. In some cases, the mixture can cause life-threatening complications. That's why it's essential that you tell your doctor about every medicine you're currently taking. And don't swallow any new medication without first talking with your doctor.

Here are some (but not all) commonly used drugs and other substances that don't mix well with blood pressure medications:

Anti-inflammatory drugs

This group of drugs includes aspirin, ibuprofen (Advil, Motrin-IB), ketoprofen (Actron, Orudis-KT), naproxen sodium (Aleve, Naprosyn), indomethacin (Indocin), and piroxicam (Feldene). They can increase the amount of salt and water retained by your body, thus interfering with diuretics. They can also impede the ability of beta blockers and ACE inhibitors to work.

What to do. Studies indicate that if you're taking high blood pressure medications, you probably don't need to worry about the occasional use of anti-inflammatory drugs—for a headache, say, or a sore muscle. But if you need to take anti-inflammatory drugs long-term, such as for arthritis or another chronic condition from which you are suffering, then you should talk to your doctor. He or she may decide to switch you to a different medication for your high blood pressure.

Cold and allergy medications

Decongestants and nasal sprays contain the ingredients pseudoephedrine or phenylephrine, which can narrow your blood vessels, causing your blood pressure to shoot up.

What to do. Avoid cold and allergy medications that contain pseudoephedrine or phenylephrine, or use them sparingly.

Sodium in Your Medications? Maybe

Did you know that everyday over-the-counter and prescription medications may contain high levels of sodium, which can elevate blood pressure and compromise the effectiveness of your high blood pressure medication? Two tablets of Alka-Seltzer contain a whopping 521 milligrams of sodium; Bromo Seltzer has 717 milligrams. Below are other medications that contain high levels of salt:

- Laxatives
- Painkillers
- Cough medications
- Antacids
- Antibiotics
- Sedatives
- Alkalizers

Diet pills

Some appetite suppressants—or diet pills—contain phenylpropanolamine, a chemical that works against high blood pressure medication by constricting blood vessels and thus raising blood pressure.

What to do. Read medication labels. Avoid any diet pills that contain phenylpropanolamine.

Oral contraceptives

The estrogen in the Pill can elevate some women's blood pressure, sometimes enough to wipe out any gains from taking an antihypertensive.

What to do. Be sure to tell your doctor if you are using the Pill. Your doctor may switch you to another form of birth control.

> **Pressure Point:** Unlike oral contraceptives, postmenopausal hormone replacement therapy (HRT) doesn't raise blood pressure. In fact, some research shows HRT slightly lowers pressure.

Corticosteroids

These drugs, which include cortisone, prednisone, and methyl-prednisolone, are used to treat inflammatory conditions and diseases, such as asthma, arthritis, skin disorders and sports injuries. They come in many forms: tablets, inhalers, creams, drops, and even injections. Regular use of the drugs can cause your body to retain salt and water, thus interfering with the action of diuretics.

What to do. Do not use these drugs without first talking with your doctor.

Antidepressants

Certain types of antidepressants, known as tricyclic antidepressants, can interfere with some central alpha agonists, such as clonidine (Catapres) and guanethidine (Ismelin).

What to do. If you are seeing different doctors for your depression and your high blood pressure, be sure that each knows all the medications you are taking.

Stretching Your Drug Dollar

Many medications for high blood pressure are quite expensive—more than a dollar a pill for some of the newer ones. What's more, statistics compiled by the High Blood Pressure Information Center show that one in 10 patients with hypertension will need to take three or more different drugs in order to control his or her blood pressure.

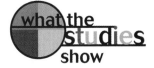

what the studies show

▶ *The 3,000-year-old Chinese medical practice of acupuncture may be helpful in lowering high blood pressure, some studies have shown. Acupuncture—a technique that involves the insertion of very thin needles into the skin to adjust the flow of energy in the body— appears to activate the body's endorphins, brain chemicals that relax muscles, dull pain, and reduce anxiety. The chemicals may also reduce blood pressure and the workload of the heart. Many doctors remain skeptical, but a study completed in 2002 could settle the question about acupuncture's role in lowering blood pressure.*

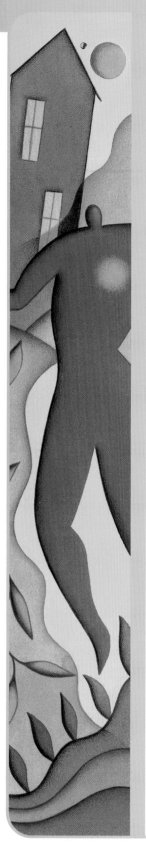

Drug Is Not a Four-Letter Word

Her whole life, Sandra Matteucci, 62, had a blood pressure to envy: 110/60 mm Hg. Two years ago, however, stress came calling and decided to stay awhile. Over five frightful months, her mother and mother-in-law died, and her husband, Ralph, sold a business, had knee and prostate-cancer surgery, and experienced blood sugar spikes that nearly killed him. To top it off, the Matteuccis bought a new house.

Her blood pressure shot up to 140-160/80-100 and stayed there long after the stress went away. She bought a relaxation book. "It didn't work," recalls Sandra, who resides in Paradise Valley, Arizona. "I tried to control things by telling myself to calm down and not let things bother me."

After six months of trying to relax, her doctor put her on medication. Sandra's blood pressure dropped to 130/80. With her doctor's approval, she went off medication for three months. Her blood pressure rose to 150/90, and she resumed taking medication. "I did not want to have a stroke, because my father had had one and died from it," she says.

Sandra has not given up on giving up blood pressure pills. She grew up in a family that tended to tough out most ailments without medication, an approach encouraged by their no-nonsense doctor.

This spring, Sandra went to the Pritikin Longevity Center in Santa Monica, California. To help her lose 10 pounds, the center established an exercise program of walking, biking, and doing strength training five days a week. She has changed her diet and her thinking about certain foods. "I love fat," she says. "God didn't give me the taste buds for broccoli and okra. But I am giving it my best shot. It's hard, but I am not going to keep putting poison in my mouth when I am trying to take care of my health."

Sandra says she is grateful she can continue taking medication until she's able to control her hypertension with diet and exercise. "Blood pressure drugs are like a lot of wonderful medications available to us—they are saving lives."

> **Sandra took drugs because she didn't want to have a stroke.**

There are several things you can do, however, to lower those expenses without putting your health in jeopardy.

Sample some samples. If you are being prescribed medications for the first time, ask your doctor for samples. This allows you time to adjust your dose, evaluate response, and monitor for side effects to the drug before investing your money.

Ask for a refill. When you are given a prescription, ask your provider to allow refills. Refills will avoid the expense of additional doctor visits just to get a prescription written.

Cutting coupons.. Ask your doctor, nurse, or pharmacist for coupons they frequently receive from drug sales representatives. Or write the drug company for coupons.

Go generic. Doctors do not always prescribe a less expensive generic drug first. Talk to your doctor about the possibility of using one. Explain that you want the most effective drug at the best price.

Shop around. Drugstores charge widely different prices for the same drugs, so get on the phone and do some comparative shopping before handing over your prescription to a pharmacist. Ask if the drugstore has a frequent buyer program or offers discount cards. If you're eligible for membership in the AARP (aged 50 or older) you might think about purchasing (for a modest annual fee) their drug discount card. It's good for savings at more than 44,000 pharmacies nationwide.

Buying in bulk. If you're going to be taking a medication for a long time, consider buying through one of the mail-order pharmacies, which often charge lower prices than their brick-and-mortar counterparts. Mail-order drug prices are usually 10 to 35 percent cheaper than prices at local pharmacies.

Do the splits. Higher-dose pills often cost only slightly more than lower-dose ones. So buying your medications at twice the strength you need and then splitting each tablet in half may save you considerable money. Talk to your doctor or pharmacist.

Ask for help. Pharmaceutical companies have programs in which they offer medications free or at a low cost to people who are faced with financial hardship. Ask your doctor to help you sign up for one of these programs. Social service agencies in your area may also help you get financial assistance to pay for your medications. Ask your doctor about these programs.

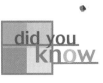

Doctors may one day be able to tailor your high blood pressure medications to fit your specific genetic makeup. Scientists took a step in that direction early in 2001 when they reported that people who have two copies of a specific gene—GNB3—responded much better to the diuretic hydrochlorothiazide than people without the gene. The scientists are now looking for other genes that may affect how well different antihypertensives work in the body.

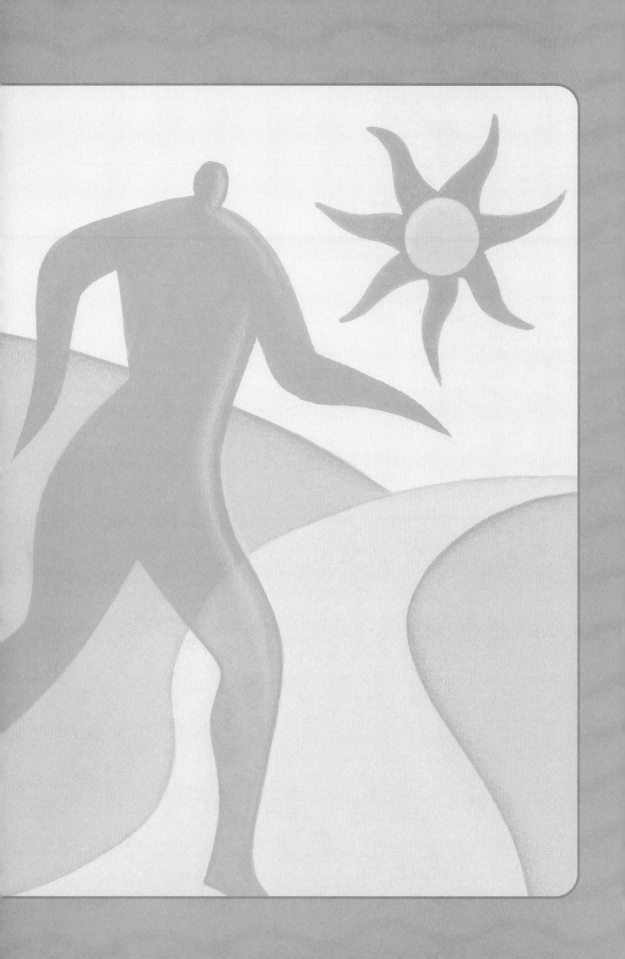

8 Staying the Course

You are gaining more than lower blood

pressure when you follow the strategies in this

book. You are improving your overall health

profile. Chances are you will live longer and

better, and reap daily rewards from sticking

with the program—like fitting into a size 8

and increasing your physical and mental energy.

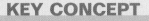

Two steps forward, one step back—expect the occasional relapse when making lifestyle changes, but don't take your eye off the long-term goal.

Accentuate the Positive

As you most certainly know by now, high blood pressure is a stealth condition. It's serious and even life-threatening, but it has no obvious symptoms. Little wonder, then, that many people with high blood pressure find it a bear to change their lifestyle and stick with their medications, day in and day out.

Of course, after reading this book you know that if you don't take charge of your high blood pressure now, you're going to have to pay the price later—recuperating, for example, from a heart attack or stroke (if you survive one of these events, that is) or dealing with kidney failure or blindness.

Sweat equity. Still, you say, it's difficult to break old, familiar (and, let's face it, often enjoyable) habits over some doom-and-gloom prediction about what might happen to you sometime in the future. You want immediate gratification for your efforts—some positive evidence that the sweat equity you're putting into your lifestyle changes is actually paying off right now.

Fair enough. Here, then, are just some of the rewards you can reap within days or weeks of adopting and faithfully following the "Low-Pressure Action Plan" outlined in chapter 1 and discussed in detail throughout this book.

The Hypertension Mind Set

Learning that you have hypertension can have side effects. A diagnosis of high blood pressure can be an acknowledgment of fact or can seem like a verdict that leaves you feeling overwhelmed. Here are some typical reactions to hypertension. Do any of them remind you of yourself?

1. **Denial.** The patient feels well and refuses to believe that anything could possibly be wrong. He or she rejects the medical findings and fails to return to the doctor who made the diagnosis.
2. **Blame.** Some people blame their job, boss, or an outside person rather than taking action to lower their blood pressure.
3. **Paralyzed by fear.** Some people who have received a diagnosis of high blood pressure become haunted by the fear that they will die or that their children will be similarly afflicted.
4. **Worry.** Other patients become worried about their general health and seek constant reassurance that they will be okay.
5. **Taking action.** Finally, some people consider a diagnosis of high blood pressure as a call to action and start making changes in their lifestyle that will help correct the condition. This group has the best chance of managing their condition.

> You'll have more energy.

> Your mood will improve.

> You'll sleep better.

> You'll be able to think more clearly.

> Your sex life will improve.

> You'll feel more relaxed and better able to deal with stress.

> You'll be able to fit back into clothes you haven't worn for years.

> And your blood pressure will go down.

Be mindful of these rewards as you work toward your goal of lowering your blood pressure. You might even want to copy the list and tape it to a mirror or your refrigerator or some other conspicuous place. Focusing on what you're gaining (all of the benefits listed on the previous page) rather than on what you're giving up (such as cigarettes and salty foods) is a great way of staying motivated—and of reaching your goals.

Finding the Motivation

We all know that change is a lot easier said than done. A lot easier. How do you get—and stay—motivated to make behavioral changes? Here are some solid tips from the experts:

Never stop learning

The more you understand about high blood pressure, the more you'll know why it's so vital to get it under control—and the

Late-Breaking News: Studies You Should Know About

Here are descriptions of two large high blood pressure trials whose final results will be reported within the next few years— results that may affect your treatment.

ALLHAT (Antihypertensive and Lipid-Lowering Treatment to Prevent Heart Attack Trial). Sponsored by the National Institutes of Health's National Heart, Lung, and Blood Institute (NHLBI), this study is being conducted in approximately 600 physicians' offices and clinics throughout the United States, Puerto Rico, the Virgin Islands, and in Canada. One of the goals of the study is to determine whether newer types of antihypertensive drugs, which are generally more costly to purchase, are as effective as diuretics in lowering the risk for heart disease.

AASK (African American Study of Kidney Disease and Hypertension). This seven-year national trial, sponsored by the National Institute of Diabetes, Digestive, and Kidney Diseases, is the first major study of kidney disease among African Americans. It hopes to answer two basic questions: What is the best level of blood pressure for preventing kidney damage? And which of three types of medication (a beta blocker, a calcium channel blocker, or an ACE inhibitor) is best for the treatment of high blood pressure in African Americans? The study will be completed in 2002.

more likely you'll stay motivated to do so. Reading *Taking Charge of High Blood Pressure* is a good first step in that learning process. But stay informed. Follow the latest news about high blood pressure in newspapers, magazines, and on the Internet, and consult the resources in the back of this book. Continue to ask your doctor questions during visits.

Think short-term

Your long-term goal is, of course, to lower your blood pressure to normal levels. That is a realistic goal. But it's not realistic to think you'll reach that goal all at once or that you can reverse a lifetime of unhealthful habits overnight. Change, unfortunately, is a lot more difficult than that.

To make permanent lifestyle changes—ones that stick—set a series of short-term goals. Take exercise, for example. If you've been a couch potato for the past 20 years, don't set a goal of running three miles by the end of the week. Instead, set up a walking schedule and then gradually add running to it. Establish weekly time and distance goals—realistic ones that you can meet. By giving yourself short-term goals (adding 10 minutes each week to a daily walk/run) as well as long-term goals (running three miles), you'll experience quicker success and thus stay motivated to continue making healthful changes.

Believe in yourself

Researchers have found that people who believe they will succeed at a particular activity are more likely to stick with it. So your success at changing your behavior depends not only on your knowing that such action will help lower your blood pressure and benefit your health but also on your belief that you can actually do it.

If you're short on self-confidence—maybe because you've failed at making major lifestyle changes before—look to others for inspiration. Find someone who has accomplished what you're trying to do and use him or her as a role model. Find out how the person went about changing his or her daily habits; ask what worked and what didn't. Borrow from the person's experience whatever you think will help you. Talking to others who have succeeded at adopting healthful behaviors can give you the knowledge and the confidence to succeed.

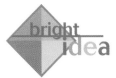

bright idea

▶ *To help yourself drop a bad, old habit, maintain a special journal for a week or two. Whenever you drink too much, eat the wrong foods, light up a cigarette, or whatever other behavior you're trying to stop, jot down the circumstances. Where were you? Who were you with? How were you feeling? And so on. After a few days, you should be able to recognize the cues that usually trigger your behavior.*

> **Pressure Point:** Make your goals SMART: Simple, Measurable, Attainable, Realistic, and Time-oriented.

Make it a group effort

Going it alone is the hardest way to undergo change. You'll be much more successful at making major lifestyle changes if you work at them with others. For inspiration and perhaps perspiration, join a walking club, a weight-loss support group, or a weekly yoga class. Or form your own "let's get healthy" support group with friends.

Baby Steps to Better Health

Goals are best achieved in a series of small, easy-to-accomplish steps. Here are some examples:

If you want to gain knowledge: "I'll go to the library for an hour this week and read more about my blood pressure medications." "I'll search the Internet for some more DASH-like menus."

If you want to exercise more: "I'll do three more sit-ups and three more push-ups this week than I did last week." "I'll increase my walking time by 10 minutes a day each week during the next month."

If you want to cut back on salt: "I won't add salt to any meals this week." "I'll purchase 'salt-free' substitutes for three packaged foods I normally eat."

If you want to lose weight: "I'll keep a journal this week of everything that I eat." "I'll cook three DASH meals this week." "I'll switch from whole milk to low-fat milk."

If you want social support: "I'll sign up for a low-fat cooking class." "I'll set three walking dates with a friend this week."

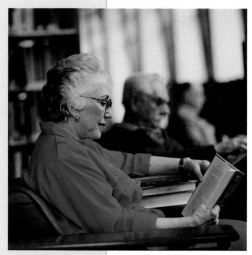

The support of your family, especially those you live with, can also be vital. Family members need to understand how important it is for you to lower your blood pressure (have them read this book!) and to be enthusiastic and supportive of your efforts to reach that goal. If you don't have familial support, however, don't give up on your efforts to get your blood pressure under control. Find others who will give you that support and continue working toward your goals.

Expect setbacks

If you have a setback in your attempts to make healthful changes in your life—and, rest assured, you will—don't treat it like a death sentence. Look at it as a problem to be solved. Figure out what caused the setback and make a plan for how you'll deal with it in the future. Make sure you don't fall into the "all-or-nothing" mental trap. Splurging on fatty fast foods at lunch doesn't mean you should abandon your healthful eating plan for the rest of the day or week. Slacking off from exercising for a few days doesn't mean you should become a permanent couch potato again.

When you slip up and fall back into old, unhealthful habits, forgive yourself. Then regroup, recharge, and re-motivate yourself! Having high blood pressure is a life-long condition. What's important is not what you do—or don't do—on a particular day, but what you accomplish day in, day out, for the rest of your life.

Sticking with the Program

Successfully managing your high blood pressure depends on your day-to-day choices and your ability to stick with your treatment program. How do you answer the following questions: Do I have to go to the gym today for a workout? Isn't it okay to skip my high blood pressure medication just this once?

Some people have an easier time than others resisting temptation and making healthful choices day in and day out, week after week, month after month. After interviewing more than 700 people, Matthew Weir of the University of Maryland Medical Center in Baltimore found that people with high blood pressure tend to fall into four distinct groups based on their ability (or inability) to control their high blood pressure. Which group do you fit in?

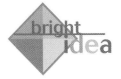

▶ *To help yourself start new, healthful habits, sit down and make a list of all the barriers in your life that have kept you from doing the desired behaviors. Now divide your list into two columns: "Can Control" and "Can't Control." You'll probably be surprised to find that most of your barriers will fall under the "Can Control" column. Come up with ways you can eliminate or minimize those barriers. If you have trouble with this brainstorming process, enlist the help of a nonjudgmental friend or family member.*

Group A: People in this group are able to control their high blood pressure through a combination of lifestyle changes and medication. Some prefer adopting healthful habits to control their BP, while others tend to rely more heavily on their medications, but all are willing to do both, if necessary.

Group B: People here depend mostly on medication for control of their blood pressure. They are very good about taking their meds as prescribed and may make some effort at lifestyle changes. Members of this group, however, are more likely to smoke and drink than Group A and less likely to exercise.

Group C: These people frequently forget to take their medications. Although they tend not to smoke or drink, they are often obese and have trouble complying with lifestyle changes.

Group D: Made up mostly of men, this group is least likely to take their blood pressure medication. If they do start on their meds, there's a good chance they'll change or stop taking the drugs without telling their doctor. People in this group are also most likely to smoke and least likely to control their diet.

Not surprisingly, Dr. Weir's research showed that people in Groups A and B have much better health outcomes than those in the other two groups. The optimum group to be in, of course, is Group A—the one in which people are actively committed to adopting healthful habits and to taking any needed medications.

> **Pressure Point:** More than a third of the people with high blood pressure believe that their blood pressure is under control when it isn't.

For many people, however, getting into Group A can seem like an insurmountable task, especially if you've already spent much of your life struggling to accomplish just one healthful change, like losing weight, exercising, or quitting smoking. Now, because of your high blood pressure, you're being told you have to make a bunch of changes—lose weight, quit smoking, alter your diet, reduce stress, and so on—and each one seems like its own Mount Everest.

How in the world can you successfully scale all those treacherous mountains? By taking it one step (or stage) at a time. Read on.

Changing Your Habits for Good

Change is a process with several distinct stages. Each is important because it helps ready us for the next one. Contrary to what you may think, change doesn't begin with action. You're unlikely to be successful for very long by turning long-held habits upside-down overnight. (Most New Year's resolutions, after all, fizzle out as fast as uncorked champagne.) You need to prepare yourself for important change, if you want the change to stick, that is.

Behavioral psychologist James Prochaska has identified and named six stages of the change process. The key to your future success at lowering your blood pressure could be as simple as determining which stage you're in and setting appropriate goals. Here is a description of each stage and strategies for progressing through them:

Stage 1: Precontemplation

When you're at this stage, you have no intention of making a change any time soon—at least not within the next six months. You may be unaware of the need to change, or you may have tried to change many times before and become demoralized by your inability to succeed at it. You tend to be in denial—you don't want to read, talk, or even think about the link between your lifestyle behaviors and your health problem (in this case, your high blood pressure). Because you cannot fail in this stage, you feel safe not taking any action.

Strategies for moving on. Because you don't (or won't) recognize that your high blood pressure is a problem, you may find it difficult to move on from this stage. Gentle, caring advice from friends and family may help you become aware of the need for change, but it's more likely that you'll raise your own consciousness about the matter, perhaps as a result of something you've read (this book!) or heard (news of a friend's heart attack). You may, of course, be catapulted into an awareness of your problem—and out of this stage—by your own heart attack or stroke.

Stage 2: Contemplation

You recognize and accept the fact that you have a health situation that needs to be changed. You're aware of all the pros of changing, but you're also very much aware of the cons. So although you plan on changing soon—at least within the next six months—you're also feeling pretty ambivalent about it. For that reason, it's very easy to get stuck in this stage for long periods of time. You may be secretly hoping that your blood pressure will improve without any effort on your part, or you may be waiting for the "right time" to start your action plan.

Strategies for moving on. Continue to raise your consciousness. Read as much as you can about the benefits of lowering blood pressure and adopting a more healthful lifestyle. Try to find and talk to other people who have successfully done it. Make a list of the "cons" of continuing with your current behavior patterns. Then list the "pros" that you can expect if you change your ways. Be specific.

Stage 3: Preparation

At this stage, you're planning to take immediate action to change your lifestyle, at least within the next month. You've made specific plans to get started, perhaps by joining a health club, buying a low-fat cookbook, or signing up for a stop-smoking class. You're ready and excited about getting started.

Strategies for moving on. Tell other people about your plans and ask them for their support. Buy a notebook or journal in which to detail your action plan and to mark your progress.

Stage 4: Action

Now you're actually changing your behavior—cutting salt from your diet, exercising daily, losing weight, and so on. Maybe you're working on improving several behaviors or maybe you're focusing on modifying only one, but you're taking some action that can be measured. Measurement (miles walked, pounds lost) is important to ensure that change is actually occurring. Action is the busiest stage and the one most noticeable to others. It's also the one where you need to be most vigilant against relapse.

Strategies for moving on. Stay committed to change. What will sweeten the pot? Set up a system of rewards, such as buying yourself a new outfit when you've lost a certain amount of weight. Learn how to substitute a healthful behavior for an unhealthful one. Take a walk instead of lighting up a cigarette, for example. Modify your environment so it's more conducive to change, perhaps by replacing the high-fat junk food in your kitchen with low-fat goodies, for instance. Also, stay in constant touch with your support system. Having someone give you a pep talk during moments of weakness may help you avoid a relapse.

Stage 5: Maintenance

The changes you implemented in stage 4 should become common, everyday habits. You must now focus on preventing a relapse. The longer you continue in the maintenance stage, the less likely you are to relapse.

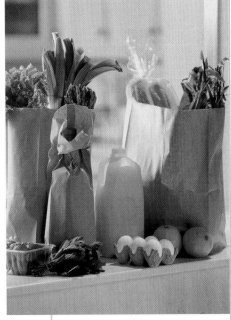

Strategies for moving on. Continue with the strategies outlined in stage 4. Avoid becoming overconfident, which can actually weaken your resolve. Make a list of all the good things that have resulted from the changes you've made. Hang up that list where you can view it often. Become a mentor for someone else who wants to change to a more healthful lifestyle. Also, continue to set new goals for yourself.

Stage 6: Termination

Not all psychologists believe anyone actually ends the process of change. Prochaska, however, believes some people can reach a point where they're no longer tempted to return to the way things were. At this stage, for example, you wouldn't even think of accepting a cigarette if someone offered it to you. Or you couldn't imagine skipping more than a day or two of exercising (and then only if you're ill or injured). Prochaska also notes, however, that few "changers"—perhaps only 20 percent—reach this stage. Some behavioral changes are more likely than others to end up here. For example, most smokers who quit eventually do reach the Termination stage.

Strategies for staying here. If you've truly terminated a behavior, you won't need any strategies because you won't be tempted to go back to your old habits. Be careful, however. You may think you've reached this stage when you're really still in Maintenance—in other words, you're still tempted by old habits, but resolved not to give in to them. So stick with the strategies outlined in stage 4. But don't forget to enjoy your success!

Relapse: Get Back on the Horse

You can revert to an earlier stage at any point in the change process. You might start preparing to exercise, for example, by signing up for a mall walking club, but then decide that your life is just too busy right now to make such a big-time commitment and, anyway, you're not quite sure you need the exercise after all. You've just slipped from stage 3 (Preparation) to stage 2 (Contemplation).

A full-blown relapse occurs when you regress from the Action or Maintenance stage to an earlier one. Relapses are quite common, so don't despair if you experience one.

> ➤**Pressure Point:** Most people cycle through the change process several times before permanently adopting a new behavior or habit.

When you have a relapse, acknowledge what has happened and work on strategies that will help you move forward again. Learn from the experience. If you started smoking again, what caused you to light up? How can you avoid that situation in the future? If you stopped exercising, ask yourself why? How can you break down those barriers?

Are You Ready for Some Changes?

A valuable tool, cumbersomely called the Readiness to Change Ruler, will help you determine if you are ready to make a lifestyle change. Behavioral experts developed it to help people who are thinking about making health-related changes, such as losing weight or cutting back on alcohol, move forward toward their goals. To find out your readiness to do the things necessary to lower your blood pressure, mark where your attitude falls on the ruler below.

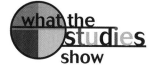

Suffering a relapse? You are not alone. According to a study conducted by Loyola University Medical Center in Chicago, only 38 percent of people who make New Year's resolutions stick to their plan a week later. After six months, the number dwindles to less than 15 percent.

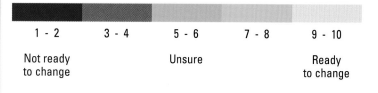

1 - 2	3 - 4	5 - 6	7 - 8	9 - 10
Not ready to change		Unsure		Ready to change

The further to the right your mark falls, the greater the possibility you'll succeed at changing your habits. But if you placed your mark somewhere to the left of "ready," don't give up on reaching your goals! You just need to do a little preliminary work to help slide yourself over into the "ready" box. You can begin answering the questions below that apply to you.

The Evolution of Change

Here are the mental shifts you will make as prospective lifestyle changes take root:

- "I'm not going to think about it."

- "I'll weigh the pros and cons."

- "I'll try a few changes and figure out how to cope with the really tough parts."

- "I'm doing it!"

- "I've made the commitment to change part of my life."

One to Two

Why do you think you're not ready to adopt a more healthful lifestyle?

What needs to happen for you to start thinking about changing?

What steps can you take to make at least one of those things happen? Put those steps in the order that you would need to do them. Mark down the date that you'll get started on the first step.

Three to Five

Why would change be good for you? Be specific.

What are the barriers that are keeping you from changing?

What steps do you need to take to overcome just one of those barriers? Put those steps in the order that you would need to do them. Mark down the date that you'll get started on the first step.

Six to Nine

What lifestyle changes have you already made?

Which of those are working? Which ones aren't?

What could you do differently to make all your efforts at change succeed?

A Perfect 10

Congratulations! What's helping you make and maintain the changes?

What else would help you?

What situations put you at risk of falling back into old, unhealthful habits?

How can you help yourself avoid those situations? Be specific.

You Are the Man (Or Woman)!

Yes, high blood pressure is a serious disease. Yes, it has no cure. And yes, you're going to have to deal with it for the rest of your life. On the other hand, you are more in charge of your health than you realize. You have the power to ensure that the outcome of controlling your high blood pressure is positive.

> ➢**Pressure Point:** If you follow the strategies and tips offered in this book—and follow your doctor's advice—chances are you can feel just as good and have the same life expectancy as your peers without high blood pressure.

Remember, there's a wealth of good news about this condition: It's highly treatable—probably the most treatable of all chronic conditions. And the treatment, which consists mostly of getting yourself (finally!) in shape, will enrich and invigorate your life. In fact, having high blood pressure might just turn out to be the best thing that's happened to you.

Lifestyle plus medication. You'll need to do some hard work, of course. You'll have to toss out some of your "bad" old habits and adopt new, healthful ones. You may have to take medications as well. And there's plenty of optimism on the medication front: Along with nine classes of antihypertensive drugs already being prescribed, there are seven new classes currently being researched: potassium channel openers, serotonin-related agents, dopamine agonists, renin inhibitors, imidazolines, neural endopeptidase inhibitors, and endothe-lin-receptor antagonists.

The more, the better. The end result is that you will have an even better chance of lowering your BP numbers with the introduction of these drugs. Two people can have the same degree of blood pressure elevation, but for two very different reasons. Each needs a BP medication that will treat the under-lying cause of his or her high blood pressure. The greater the variety of medications available, the more likely it is that the appropriate drug for the appropriate person will be found. After all, high blood pressure can be stubborn at times, so don't be surprised if you feel discouraged periodically. Just be patient and persevere.

You *can* take charge of your high blood pressure. The payoff is huge: a long, healthy, and active life. Now, wrapping your mind around that rather large payoff, is there any reason you can come up with that can possibly justify not taking charge of your condition—today, now. We didn't think so.

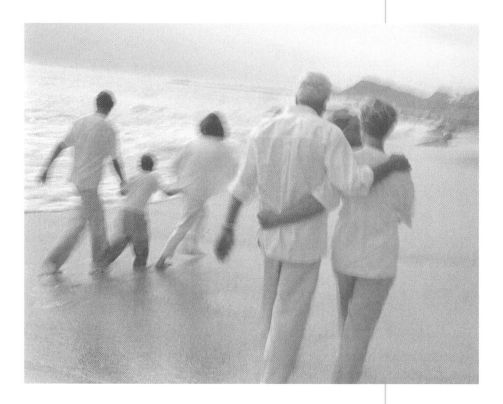

Helpful Organizations and Associations

If you need more information about high blood pressure and related conditions—or help in making lifestyle changes—here are some solid places to start.

Hypertension and the Heart

American Heart Association
7272 Greenville Avenue
Dallas, TX 75231
214-373-6300
800-AHA-USA1
www.americanheart.org

American Society of Hypertension
515 Madison Ave., Suite 1212
New York, NY 10022
212-644-0650
www.ash-us.org

Hypertension Network
www.bloodpressure.com

National Heart, Lung, and Blood Institute
Information Center
P.O. Box 30105
Bethesda, MD 20824-0105
800-575-WELL
www.nih.gov/health/consumer/conicd.htm

National Hypertension Association
324 East 30th St.
New York, NY 10016
212-889-3557
www.nathypertension.org

Lifestyle Changes

Alcoholics Anonymous World Services
P.O. Box 459, Grand Central Station
New York, NY 10163
212-870-3400
www.aa.org

American Lung Association [for help with quitting smoking]
1740 Broadway
New York, NY 10019
800-LUNG-USA (800-586-4872)
www.lungusa.org

DASH Diet
www.dash.bwh.harvard.edu

Mended Hearts
7272 Greenville Ave.
Dallas, TX 75231-4596
214-706-1442
www.mendedhearts.org

The Mind-Body Medical Institute
Division of Behavioral Medicine
Beth Israel Deaconess Medical Center
110 Francis St.
Boston, MA 02215
617-632-9530
www.mindbody.harvard.edu

The Weight-Control Information Network
1 WIN Way
Bethesda, MD 20892-3665
202-828-1025
877-946-4627
www.niddk.nih.gov/health/nutrit/win.htm

Related Conditions

American Diabetes Association
1701 N. Beauregard St.
Alexandria, VA 22311
800-232-3472
www.diabetes.org

National Diabetes Information
Clearinghouse (NDIC)
1 Information Way
Bethesda, MD 20892-3560
301-654-3327
800-860-8747
www.niddk.nih.gov

National Eye Institute
31 Center Dr.
Bethesda, MD 20892-2510
301-496-5248
www.nei.nih.gov

National Kidney and Urologic Diseases
Information Clearinghouse (NKUDIC)
3 Information Way
Bethesda, MD 20892-3580
301-654-4415
800-891-5390
www.niddk.nih.gov

National Institute of Neurological Disorders
and Stroke
P.O. Box 5801
Bethesda, MD 20824
800-352-9424
www.ninds.nih.gov

National Kidney Foundation
30 East 33rd St., Suite 1100
New York, NY 10016
800-622-9010
www.kidney.org

National Stroke Association
9707 East Easter Lane
Englewood, CO 80112-3747
800-STROKES (800-787-6537)
www.stroke.org

Alternative Medicine

National Center for Complementary and
Alternative Medicine Clearinghouse
P.O. Box 8218
Silver Spring, MD 20907-8218
888-644-6226
www.nccam.nih.gov

Miscellaneous

Centers for Disease Control
www.cdc.gov

Healthfinder
www.healthfinder.gov

National Institute on Aging
Information Center
P.O. Box 8057
Gaithersburg, MD 20898-8057
800-222-2225
800-222-4225 (TTY)
www.aoa.dhhs.gov/aoa

National Women's Health Network
514 10th St. NW, Suite 400
Washington, DC 20004
202-628-7814
www.womenshealthnetwork.org

High Blood Pressure Drugs: At A Glance

Generic Drug	Brand Name	Dose	Relative Cost
Thiazide diuretics			
Chlorthalidone	Hygroton, Thalidone	12.5 to 50 mg/ once per day	$$$
Hydrochlorothiazide	Esidrix, HydroDiuril, Oretic, Microzide	12.5 to 50 mg/ once a day	$$$
Hydroflumethiazide	Diucardin	25 to 200 mg/ once a day	$$
Indapamide	Lozol	1.25 to 5 mg/ once a day	$$$$
Methyclothiazide	Enduron, Aquatensen	2.5 to 10 mg/ once a day	$$
Metolazone	Mykrox, Zaroxolyn	0.5 to 1 mg/ once a day (Mykrox); 2.5 to 10 mg / once a day (Zaroxolyn)	$$$
Polythiazide	Renese	1 to 4 mg/ once a day	$$
Loop diuretics			
Bumetanide	Bumex	0.5 to 4 mg/ 2 to 3 times a day	$
Furosemide	Lasix	20 to 480 mg/ 2 to 3 times a day	$$
Torsemide	Demadex	5 to 40 mg / 1 to 2 times a day	$$
Potassium-sparing diuretics			
Amiloride hydrochloride	Midamor	5 to 10 mg/ once a day	$$
Spironolactone	Aldactone	25 to 100 mg/ once a day	$$$
Beta blockers			
Acebutolol hydrochloride	Sectral	200 to 800/ once a day	$$$$ $$

Diuretics: Capsule Summary

Advantages: Diuretics have been proven effective and safe for lowering blood pressure; they are also relatively inexpensive. Thus, they are often the first drug of choice for treating hypertension. Loop diuretics are sometimes recommended for people with congestive heart failure or other conditions that cause the body to retain fluid.

Disadvantages: Diuretics can cause frequent urination, fatigue, dizziness on standing, impotence, increased sensitivity to sunlight, gout, dehydration, and small increases in blood sugar and cholesterol. High doses of thiazide diuretics (50 to 100 milligrams per day) may increase the risk for heart attacks. Thiazide and loop diuretics can cause the body to lose too much potassium. Potassium-sparing diuretics raise potassium levels, which can be dangerous for people with kidney disease. Caution should be taken when using potassium-sparing diuretics with ACE inhibitors, which also raise potassium levels.

Beta Blockers: Capsule Summary

Advantages: Along with diuretics, these drugs are frequently chosen as the first line of treatment for high blood pressure. They

continued on next page

Note: Talk with your doctor first before making any changes in dosage or switching prescriptions.

Generic Drug	Brand Name	Dose	Relative Cost
Atenolol	Tenormin	25 to 100 mg/ 1 to 2 times a day	$$$$
Betaxolol hydrochloride	Kerlone	5 to 20 mg/ once a day	$$$
Bisoprolol fumarate	Zebeta	2.5 to 10 mg/ once a day	$$$$$
Carvedilol	Coreg	2.5 to 50 mg/ once a day	$$$$$
Carteolol hydrochloride	Cartrol	2.5 to 10 mg/ once a day	$$$$
Labetalol	Normodyne, Trandate	200 to1200 mg/ once a day	$$$
Metoprolol tartrate	Lopressor	50 to 300 mg/ 2 times a day	$$$$
Metoprolol succinate	Toprol XL	50 to 300 mg/ once a day	$$$$ $$
Penbutolol sulfate	Levatol	10 to 20 mg/ once a day	$$$$$
Pindolol	Visken	10 to 60 mg/ 2 times a day	$$$$$ $$$
Propranolol	Inderal	40 to 480 mg/ once a day	$$$$$
Propranolol hydrochloride	Inderal LA	40 to 480 mg/ 2 times a day	$$$$$ $$$
Timolol maleate	Blocadren	20 to 60 mg/ 2 times a day	$$$
ACE inhibitors			
Benazepril hydrochloride	Lotensin	5 to 40 mg/ 1 to 2 times a day	$$$
Captopril	Capoten	25 to 150 mg/ 2 to 3 times a day	$$$$$ $$
Enalapril maleate	Vasotec	5 to 40 mg/ 1 to 2 times a day	$$$$
Fosinopril sodium	Monopril	10 to 40 mg/ 1 to 2 times a day	$$$

Beta Blockers *(continued from p. 240)*

have characteristics that also make them helpful for people with angina or an arrhythmia or who have had a prior heart attack.

Disadvantages: Fatigue is the most common side effect of these drugs, so active people may want to avoid them. Because these drugs can weaken the heart and constrict airways, they also should be avoided by people with congestive heart failure and lung diseases, such as asthma and emphysema. People with diabetes should be cautious about using these drugs, which can mask drops in blood sugar levels.

ACE Inhibitors: Capsule Summary

Advantages: These drugs cause few side effects. They are good for active people because they don't produce fatigue. The drugs also may slow kidney damage in people with diabetes. Unlike diuretics and beta blockers, ACE inhibitors don't raise blood cholesterol, which makes them a good choice for people with high cholesterol. Ramipril has been shown to lower the risk for heart attack, stroke, and diabetes.

Disadvantages: Many people using these drugs develop a dry cough. A few develop a

continued on next page

Generic Drug	Brand Name	Dose	Relative Cost
Lisinopril	Prinivil, Zestril	5 to 40 mg/ once a day	$$$
Moexipril hydrochloride	Univasc	25 to 100 mg/ 1 to 2 times a day	$$$
Perindopril erbumine	Aceon	2 to 16 mg/ once a day or divided doses	$$$$
Quinapril hydrochloride	Accupril	5 to 80 mg/ 1 to 2 times a day	$$$$
Ramipril	Altace	1.25 to 20 mg/ 1 to 2 times a day	$$$$
Trandolapril	Mavik	1 to 4 mg/ once a day	$$$
Angiotensin II receptor blockers			
Candesartan cilexetil	Atacand	4 to 32 mg/ 1 or 2 times a day	$$$$$
Irbesarten	Avapro	150 to 300 mg/ once a day	$$$$$
Lorsartin potassium	Cozaar	25 to 100 mg/ 1 or 2 times a day	$$$$$
Valsartan	Diovan	80 to 320 mg/ once a day	$$$$$
Calcium channel blockers (long-acting)			
Amlodipine besylate	Norvasc	2.5 to 10 mg/ once a day	$$$$$
Diltiazem	Cardizem CD, Cardizem SR, Dilacor XR, Tiazac	120 to 360 mg/ once a day; 2 times a day (Cardizem SR)	$$$$$ $
Felodipine	Plendil	2.5 to 20 mg/ once a day	$$$$
Isradipine	DynaCirc, DynaCirc CR	5 to 20 mg/ once a day (DynaCirc CR); 2 times a day (DynaCirc)	$$$$$ $

Note: Talk with your doctor first before making any changes in dosage or switching prescriptions.

ACE Inhibitors *(continued from p. 241)*

skin rash, swelling in the mouth, or a lessening of their ability to taste. People with severe kidney disease must use these drugs with caution. Pregnant women should avoid these drugs as should other women of childbearing years, unless they are using effective contraception.

Angiotensin II Receptor Blockers: Capsule Summary

Advantages: These drugs have few side effects. They work similar to ACE inhibitors, but don't produce a cough and need to be taken only once a day. Lorsartin has been shown to improve hypertension-related male impotence.

Disadvantages: Although uncommon, side effects can include dizziness and fatigue. Pregnant and breastfeeding women should avoid these drugs. So should women in their childbearing years, unless they are using effective contraception.

Calcium Channel Blockers (long-acting): Capsule Summary

Advantages: Side effects of these drugs tend to be mild. Because they do not produce fatigue, they are sometimes recommended for active people. These drugs have proven especially effective in African Americans and older people.

Disadvantages: Possible side effects include constipation, a rapid heartbeat, dizziness, nausea, and swelling, especially of the feet, lower legs, and gums. These drugs should be used cautiously by people with heart arrhythmia or liver disease.

continued on next page

Generic Drug	Brand Name	Dose	Relative Cost
Nicardipine hydrochloride	Cardene SR	60 to 90 mg/ 2 times a day	$$$$$
Nifedipine	Adalat CC, Procardia XL	30 to 120 mg/ once a day	$$$$ $$$$
Nisoldipine	Sular	20 to 60 mg/ once a day	$$$
Verapamil hydrochloride	Isoptin SR, Calan SR, Verelan, Covera HS	90 to 480 mg/ 2 times a day (Isoptin SR, Calan SR) 120 to 480 mg/ once a day (Verelan, Covera HS)	$$$$ $$$
Alpha blockers			
Doxazosin mesylate	Cardura	1 to 16 mg/ once a day	$$$$
Labetalol hydrochloride	Normodyne	100 to 800 mg/ once a day	$$$$
Prazosin hydrochloride	Minipress	2 to 30 mg/ 2 to 3 times a day	$$$
Terazosin hydrochloride	Hytrin	1 to 20 mg/ once a day	$$$$ $$$
Central alpha agonists			
Clonidine hydrochloride	Catapres	0.2 to 1.2 mg/ 2 to 3 times a day	$$$
Guanabenz acetate	Wytensin	8 to 32 mg/ 2 times a day	$$$$ $$$
Guanfacine hydrochloride	Tenex	1 to 3 mg/ once a day	$$$$
Methyldopa	Aldomet	500 to 3000 mg/ 2 times a day	$$$

Calcium Channel Blockers
(continued from p. 242)

Recent studies suggest that these drugs may increase the risk for heart attack. Other studies suggest these drugs may make men temporarily infertile.

Alpha Blockers: Capsule Summary

Advantages: These drugs are helpful for people with high cholesterol because they lower triglycerides and LDL cholesterol. They can also help reduce the symptoms of benign prostatic hyperplasia (BPH) in older men.

Disadvantages: People sometimes become very dizzy or even faint after taking these drugs, especially after the first dose. The effectiveness of the drugs can diminish over time. Recent studies have found that doxazosin may increase the risk for heart failure.

Central Alpha Agonists: Capsule Summary

Advantages: These drugs can also help ease symptoms associated with migraine headaches, panic attacks, and drug or alcohol withdrawal. Methyldopa is considered safe for use by pregnant women. Catapres is available as a skin patch that is reapplied only once a week.

Disadvantages: Severe dizziness and/or drowsiness, may occur. Other possible side effects include nausea, rapid heartbeat, headache, dry mouth, constipation, fatigue, sleep problems, depression, anxiety, and impotence.

Generic Drug	Brand Name	Dose	Relative Cost
Peripheral-acting adrenergic antagonists			
Guanadrel sulfate	Hylorel	10 to 75 mg/ 2 times a day	$$$$ $$$$
Guanethidine monosulfate	Ismelin	10 to 50 mg/ once a day	$$$$
Reserpine	Serpasil	0.05 to 0.25mg/ once a day	$$
Blood vessel dilators			
Hydralazine hydrochloride	Apresoline	50 to 300 mg/ 2 times a day	$$$$
Minoxidil	Loniten	5 to 100 mg/ once a day	$$$$$

Peripheral-Acting Adrenergic Antagonists

Advantages: These drugs can be very effective for cases of severe hypertension. Their side effects can sometimes be countered by taking them with other antihypertensives. Guanadrel sulfate and guanethidine monosulfate do not cause drowsiness. The drug Reserpine is relatively inexpensive.

Disadvantages: Guanadrel and guanethidine can cause blood pressure to quickly plunge upon standing or with exercise. Reserpine has been linked to the sudden onset of serious depression. Other possible side effects include drowsiness (reserpine only), diarrhea, dryness of mouth, loss of appetite, nausea, nasal congestion, and impotence.

Blood Vessel Dilators: Capsule Summary

Advantages: These potent drugs can be very effective in cases of severe hypertension. Side effects can be minimized by combining these drugs with a beta-blocker and a diuretic. Minoxidil is helpful when severe hypertension is accompanied by kidney problems.

Disadvantages: These drugs can speed up the heart and cause the body to retain water, which is why they are usually prescribed with other antihypertensives. Other possible side effects include dizziness, headache, loss of appetite, gastrointestinal problems, eye tearing, stuffy nose, skin rash, and breast tenderness. Minoxidil may cause body hair to grow in thicker or darker. High doses of hydralazine may increase the risk for developing lupus.

Note: Talk with your doctor first before making any changes in dosage or switching prescriptions.

DASH Meal Plan: Five Days of Healthy Eating   Day 1

2,400 mg Sodium Menu	Sodium (mg)	Substitutions to Reduce Sodium to 1,500 mg	Sodium (mg)	Number of DASH Food Group Servings							
				Grains	Vegetables	Fruits	Dairy foods	Meat, poultry & fish	Nuts, seeds, & dry beans	Fats & oils	Sweets
Breakfast											
⅔ cup bran cereal	161	⅔ cup shedded wheat cereal	124	1							
1 slice whole-wheat bread	149			1							
1 medium banana	1					1					
1 cup fruit yogurt, fat free, no sugar added	53						1				
1 cup fat-free milk	126						1				
2 tsp jelly	5										⅔
Lunch											
¾ cup chicken salad	201	No salt	127					1		1	
2 slices whole-wheat bread	299			2							
1 Tbsp Dijon mustard	372	1 Tbsp regular mustard	196								
Salad:											
½ cup fresh cucumber slices	8				1						
½ cup tomato wedges	1				1						
2 Tbsp ranch dressing, fat free	306	2 Tbsp yogurt salad dressing	84								
½ cup fruit cocktail, juice pack	5						1				
Dinner											
3 oz. beef, eye of round	52							1			
2 Tbsp beef gravy, low fat	163	2 Tbsp beef gravy, low fat, unsalted	5								
1 cup green beans, cooked from frozen	12				2						
1 small baked potato:	7				1						
2 Tbsp sour cream, fat free	28										
2 Tbsp grated cheddar cheese, natural, reduced fat	86	2 Tbsp cheddar cheese, natural, reduced fat, low sodium	1				¼				
1 Tbsp chopped scallions	1										
1 small whole-wheat roll	148			1							
1 tsp soft margarine	51	1 tsp soft margarine, unsalted	1							1	
1 small apple	0					1					
1 cup fat-free milk	126						1				
Snack											
⅓ cup almonds, unsalted	5								1		
¼ cup raisins	2					1					
1 cup orange juice	2					1⅓					
Totals				5	5	5⅓	3¼	2	1	2	⅔

Source: DASH Diet, Harvard University

Day 2

2,400 mg Sodium Menu	Sodium (mg)	Substitutions to Reduce Sodium to 1,500 mg	Sodium (mg)	Number of DASH Food Group Servings							
				Grains	Vegetables	Fruits	Dairy foods	Meat, poultry & fish	Nuts, seeds, & dry beans	Fats & oils	Sweets
Breakfast											
½ cup instant oatmeal, flavored	104	½ cup regular oatmeal, with 1 tsp cinnamon	1	1							
1 mini whole-wheat bagel	84			1							
1 medium banana	1					1					
1 cup fat-free milk	126						1				
1 Tbsp cream cheese, fat free	75										
Lunch											
Chicken breast sandwich:											
2 slices (3 oz.) chicken breast, skinless	65							1			
2 slices whole-wheat bread	299			2							
1 slice (¾ oz.) American cheese, reduced fat	328	1 slice (¾ oz.) Swiss cheese, natural	54				½				
1 large leaf romaine lettuce	1				¼						
2 slices tomato	4				½						
1 Tbsp mayonnaise, low fat	90									1	
1 medium peach	0					1					
1 cup apple juice	7					1⅓					
Dinner											
¾ cup vegetarian spaghetti sauce	459	Substitute no-salt-added tomato paste (6 oz.)	260		1½						
1 cup spaghetti	1			2							
3 Tbsp Parmesan cheese	349						½				
Spinach salad:											
1 cup fresh spinach leaves	24				1						
¼ cup fresh carrots, grated	10				½						
¼ cup fresh mushrooms, sliced	1				½						
2 Tbsp vinaigrette dressing	0									¾	
½ cup corn, cooked from frozen	4				1						
½ cup canned pears, juice packed	4					1					
Snack											
⅓ cup almonds	5								1		
¼ cup dried apricots	3					1					
1 cup fruit yogurt, fat free, no sugar added	107						1				
Totals				6	5¼	5⅓	3	1	1	1¾	0

2,400 mg Sodium Menu	Sodium (mg)	Substitutions to Reduce Sodium to 1,500 mg	Sodium (mg)	Number of DASH Food Group Servings							
				Grains	Vegetables	Fruits	Dairy foods	Meat, poultry & fish	Nuts, seeds, & dry beans	Fats & oils	Sweets
Breakfast											
¾ cup wheat flakes cereal	199	2 cups puffed wheat cereal	1	1							
1 slice whole-wheat bread	149			1							
1 medium banana	1					1					
1 cup fat-free milk	126						1				
1 cup orange juice	5					1⅓					
1 tsp soft margarine	51	1 tsp soft margarine, unsalted	1							1	
Lunch											
Beef barbecue sandwich:											
2 oz. beef, eye of round	35							⅔			
1 Tbsp barbecue sauce	156										
2 slices (1½ oz.) cheddar cheese, reduced fat	260	2 slices (1½ oz.) Swiss cheese, natural	109				1				
1 sesame roll	319			1							
1 large leaf romaine lettuce	1				¼						
2 slices tomato	22				½						
1 cup new potato salad	12				2						
1 medium orange	0					1					
Dinner											
3 oz. cod:	89							1			
1 tsp lemon juice	1										
½ cup brown rice, long grain	5			1							
½ cup spinach, cooked from frozen	88				1						
1 small corn bread muffin	363	1 small white dinner roll	146	1							
1 tsp soft margarine	51	1 tsp soft margarine, unsalted	1							1	
Snack											
1 cup fruit yogurt, fat free, no added sugar	107						1				
¼ cup dried fruit	6					1					
2 large graham cracker rectangles	156			1							
1 Tbsp peanut butter, reduced fat	101	1 Tbsp peanut butter, unsalted	3						½		
Totals				6	3¾	4⅓	3	1⅔	½	2	0

Day 4

2,400 mg Sodium Menu	Sodium (mg)	Substitutions to Reduce Sodium to 1,500 mg	Sodium (mg)	Number of DASH Food Group Servings							
				Grains	Vegetables	Fruits	Dairy foods	Meat, poultry & fish	Nuts, seeds, & dry beans	Fats & oils	Sweets
Breakfast											
¾ cup cornflakes	223	½ cup corn grits, with 1 tsp nonfat margarine, unsalted	1 1	1							
½ cup fruit yogurt, fat free, no added sugar	53						½				
1 medium apple	0					1					
1 cup grape juice	8					1 ⅓					
1 cup fat-free milk	126						1				
Lunch											
Ham and cheese sandwich:											
2 oz. smoked ham, low fat, low sodium	469	2 oz. roast beef, low fat	35					⅔			
1 slice (¾ oz.) cheddar cheese, natural, reduced fat	130						½				
2 slices whole-wheat bread	299			2							
1 large leaf romaine lettuce	1				¼						
2 slices tomato	22				½						
1 Tbsp mayonnaise, low fat	90									1	
1 cup carrot sticks	43				2						
Dinner											
Chicken and spanish rice	367	Substitute no-salt-added tomato sauce (4 oz.)	226	1				1			
½ cup green peas, cooked from frozen	70				1						
1 cup cantaloupe	14					2					
1 small whole-wheat roll	148			1							
1 cup fat-free milk	126						1				
1 tsp soft margarine	51	1 tsp soft margarine, unsalted	1							1	
Snack											
⅓ cup almonds, unsalted	5								1		
½ cup fruit cocktail	5					1					
1 cup apple juice	7					1 ⅓					
Totals				5	3 ¾	6 ⅔	3	1 ⅔	1	2	0

2,400 mg Sodium Menu	Sodium (mg)	Substitutions to Reduce Sodium to 1,500 mg	Sodium (mg)	Number of DASH Food Group Servings							
				Grains	Vegetables	Fruits	Dairy foods	Meat, poultry & fish	Nuts, seeds, & dry beans	Fats & oils	Sweets
Breakfast											
¾ cup frosted shredded wheat	3			1							
2 slices whole-wheat bread	299			2							
1 medium banana	1					1					
1 cup fat-free milk	126						1				
1 cup orange juice	5					1 ⅓					
1 tsp soft margarine	51	1 tsp soft margarine, unsalted	1							1	
2 tsp jelly, no added sugar	0										
Lunch											
Salad plate:											
½ cup tuna salad	158							1			
1 large leaf romaine lettuce	1				¼						
6 wheat crackers, fat free	107	6 wheat crackers, fat free, unsalted	18	1							
½ cup cottage cheese, 2%	459	½ cup cottage cheese, 2%, unsalted	23				¼				
1 cup canned pineapple, juice packed	2					2					
4 small celery sticks	59				½						
2 Tbsp ranch dressing, fat free	306	2 Tbsp yogurt dressing, fat free	84								
Dinner											
3 oz. turkey meatloaf	62							1			
1 Tbsp catsup	178	2 tsp catsup	119								
1 small baked potato:	7			1							
1 tsp soft margarine	51	1 tsp soft margarine, unsalted								1	
1 Tbsp sour cream, low fat	15										
1 scallion stalk, chopped	2										
1 cup collard greens, cooked from frozen	15				2						
1 medium peach	0					1					
1 cup fat-free milk	126						1				
Snack											
1 Tbsp peanut butter, reduced fat	101	1 Tbsp peanut butter, reduced fat, unsalted	3						½		
½ medium bagel (3-inch diameter)	152			1							
½ cup fruit yogurt, fat free, no added sugar	53						½				
Totals				5	3¾	5⅓	2¾	2	½	2	0

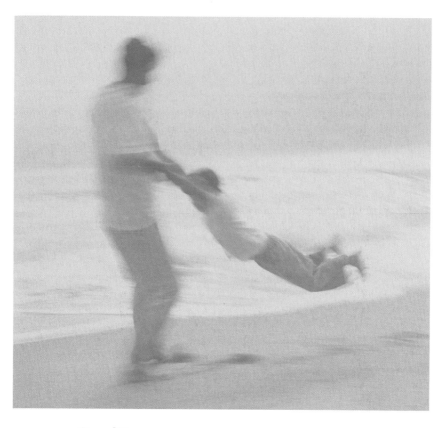

Credits

Photo
Front Cover and page 2 Will Crocker.
16 PhotoDisc. **18** PhotoDisc. **19** PhotoDisc. **20** PhotoDisc.
21 PhotoDisc. **22** PhotoDisc. **31** FDR Library and Digital Archives.
50 PhotoDisc. **52** PhotoDisc **53** *top right*: Eyewire. **53** *center and bottom right*: PhotoDisc. **64** Eyewire. **67** PhotoDisc. **69** PhotoDisc.
82 PhotoDisc. **84** PhotoDisc. **86** PhotoDisc. **94** Comstock.
95 Comstock. **103** *top right and center*: Comstock. *bottom right*:
PhotoDisc. **105** PhotoDisc. **107** PhotoDisc. **107** PhotoDisc.
111 PhotoDisc. **114** PhotoDisc. **120** Comstock. **122** PhotoDisc.
125-129 Beth Bischoff. **147** Corbis. **150** PhotoDisc. **154** Eyewire.
157 Lisa Koenig. **160** Eyewire. **165** PhotoDisc. **176** PhotoDisc.
183 Eyewire. **187** PhotoDisc. **192** Eyewire. **201** Comstock.
214 PhotoDisc. **216** Comstock. **229** PhotoDisc. **233** PhotoDisc.
237 DigitalVision. **256** DigitalVision.

Illustration
All illustrations by Tracy Walker except **39, 40** Articulate Graphics